INDIAN CLUBS

AND

HOW TO USE THEM.

A NEW AND COMPLETE METHOD FOR LEARNING TO WIELD LIGHT AND HEAVY CLUBS
GRADUATED FROM THE SIMPLEST TO THE MOST COMPLICATED EXERCISES.

BY

E. FERDINAND LEMAIRE,

FOURTEEN YEARS MEMBER AND LEADER OF THE GERMAN GYMNASTIC SOCIETY, LONDON ;
TWO YEARS HONORARY DIRECTOR OF EXERCISES OF THE AMATEUR GYMNASTIC CLUB, LONDON
AND
HONORARY MEMBER OF SEVERAL OTHER GYMNASTIC SOCIETIES.

(Winner of the Gold Medal at the Leeds All Weights Indian Clubs Open Competition, 1876.)

WITH 218 ILLUSTRATIONS BY THE AUTHOR.

FOLLOWED BY AN APPENDIX ON

STRENGTH AND STRONG MEN.

1889.

British Library Cataloguing-in-Publication Data
A catalogue record for this book is available from the
British Library

Indian Clubs

'Indian clubs', or 'Iranian clubs' belong to a category of exercise equipment used for developing strength, and in juggling. In appearance, they resemble elongated bowling-pins, and are commonly made out of wood. They come in all shapes and sizes however, ranging from a few pounds each, to fifty pounds, and are commonly swung in certain patterns as part of exercise programs. They were often used in class formats, predominantly in Iran, where members would perform choreographed routines, led by an instructor; remarkably similar to modern aerobics classes. Despite their name, 'Indian clubs' actually originated in ancient Persia, Egypt and the Middle East, where they were used by wrestlers. The practice has continued to the present day, notably in the varzesh-e bastani tradition practiced in the zurkaneh of Iran. British colonialists first came across these eastern artefacts in India however, hence the name. The 'Indian clubs' became exceedingly popular back in the UK, especially during the health craze of the Victorian era. In a book written in 1866, by an American sports enthusiast, S.D. Kehoe, it was stated that 'as a means of physical culture, the Indian Clubs stand pre-eminent among the varied apparatus of Gymnastics now in use.' He had visited England in 1861, and was so impressed with the sport that he began to manufacture and sell clubs to the American public in 1862. They were used by military cadets and upper class ladies alike, and even appeared as a gymnastic event at the 1904 and 1932

Olympics. Their popularity began to wane in the 1920s however, with the growing predilection for organised sports. The modern juggling club was inspired by the 'Indian club' though; first repurposed for juggling by DeWitt Cook in the 1800s. He taught his step son, Claude Bartram to juggle with them, who later went on to form the first 'club juggling act'. Today, their popularity has been revived somewhat, by fitness enthusiasts who that they are a far safer means of excising, rather than the traditional 'free weight regimens'. Nostalgic replicas of the original clubs are still manufactured, as well as modern engineering updates to the concept, such as the Clubbell.

CONTENTS.

PREFACE.

I DEDICATE this book to the many friends to whom I may have had, at different times, the pleasure of giving hints or more extended instruction on the use of Indian Clubs.

Having often been asked if I knew of a good book on Indian Clubs, and believing that all those treating of the subject fall far short of the ordinary requirements of anyone wishing to become proficient in that branch of athletics, I have determined to write this book, introducing in it all that my long experience has taught me. Here I may say that I have not been guided by any other book, or any other person's ideas or principles. The whole of this work is entirely original, the system I have made use of is my own invention, and the whole of the illustrations are from my own designs.

The method I have employed is based on five simple circles, which, by being gradually added and combined together, carry the learner progressively from the most simple to the most difficult exercises. I demonstrated it in public at a gymnastic display given in the Albert Hall, in connection with the Health Exhibition, by making a squad of fifty men go through over a hundred different evolutions, starting with the most simple and gradually increasing to the most intricate, and my system made a great impression on the spectators, among whom were many competent judges. The five circles I have mentioned, and which are designated by distinctive names, are in themselves extremely simple, but, although the diagrams representing them would suffice for any one to understand how to do them, I have devoted upwards of 50 pages and illustrations to their explanation, so that the student may be thoroughly familiar with them before any exercises are attempted. This method not only enables any one unacquainted with Indian Clubs to become thoroughly proficient, but it is also of the greatest value to advanced performers and teachers, as it shows them how to form exercises and combine them together. In all the illustrations the circular course of the right club is clearly distinguished from that of the left, the former being traced by dots, the latter by dashes or strokes.

The book is full of valuable hints and explanations, and comprises exercises not only for the most advanced gymnasts, but also for ladies, children, and schools; it has also a special chapter on heavy clubs. The work finishes with an appendix on Strength and Strong Men, giving a record of some wonderful feats performed by athletes and historical personages from the earliest ages to the present time.

I may as well mention that this book is not intended as a literary or artistic work, but simply as a practical handbook.

My name must be familiar to any one who may have taken an interest in athletics during the last 14 years, as for that time I have wielded the clubs at nearly 200 assaults-of-arms and gymnastic displays. As regards those who do not happen to know me, I hope they will soon be convinced that I possess the necessary qualifications for the task I have undertaken. I have practised gymnastics in general for about 25 years, and have taught Indian Clubs at the German Gymnasium and elsewhere for upwards of 12 years. I have also been the Honorary Director of Exercises of the Amateur Gymnastic Club, for two years, until its dissolution. I may say that I have shown how to use the clubs to thousands of persons, including some of the best professional teachers of the day.

Now, I think the reader will be convinced that I must know something about what I have compiled in this volume, and I trust that he will have that confidence in me which I think it is necessary the pupil should have in his teacher.

E. FERDINAND LEMAIRE

London, October, 1889.

INTRODUCTION.

INDIAN Clubs are perhaps the most ancient of the gymnastic implements used at the present time. Their use can be traced to the most remote antiquity. Persian Clubs would be a far more correct name for them, as in their present shape they were much more used by Persians than Indians. In the Tower of London can be seen a pair of clubs from India. They are made of very heavy wood, and are somewhat in the shape that I recommend further on for heavy clubs.

The Persians and Indians use their clubs principally by holding them in the reverse way from what we do in this country; that is, the club hanging below the little finger, instead of being above the thumb and first finger. Their favourite exercise consists of doing small circles above the head.

The Greeks and the Romans made great use of them, and gave them a prominent place among their various gymnastic exercises. At the present time clubs are much more used in England and America than in any other part of the world. On the Continent their use is very limited, and they are practised with more after the fashion of dumb-bells.

That the club is the most ancient weapon nobody can deny; it is also the most natural and handy that could be found, and consequently the first used by man, for we find that Cain slew Abel with a club. The ordinary weapon of the athletic god Hercules was a club; and though he also used the bow and arrow, he is always represented with his club. In ancient times, both in Greece and Rome, the strongest athletes, on public occasions, were fond of brandishing clubs, believing themselves to be representatives of Hercules. We hear of Milo of Crotona leading his compatriots to war armed with a club. A Roman emperor, Commodus, proud of his immense strength, paraded the streets with a club as Hercules.

Bacchus is said to have conquered India with an army of satyrs and bacchantes armed with clubs. Samson would have been very good with clubs when we consider what he did with a jawbone, which was simply for him a kind of club. Some theologists believe that the Samson of the Jews is the same person as the Hercules of mythology. Clubs were favourite weapons with the fighting bishops and other prelates of the early and middle ages. They thought that if they were not allowed to kill people in the ordinary way, with swords, spears, or arrows, nothing could forbid their knocking them down. We find that at all times the principal weapon of uncivilised races were and are clubs, and going still a little lower we also find that the higher races of monkeys, such as the ourang-outang, fight with branches, which they use as clubs, and travellers tell us that thus armed they are most formidable antagonists to encounter.

Thus, clubs, in one form or another, have had a conspicuous place in nature, mythology, and history. But what interests us more here is the adaptation of clubs to the development of health and strength. To those who, for certain reasons, do not care or find it impossible to go in for the head-over-heel style of gymnastics, Indian clubs are most invaluable. I shall even go further and say that, to runners, walkers, boxers, rowers, and swimmers—in fact, to anyone practising any special branch of athletics, they are also of the greatest use, as they open the chest, strengthen the back, the arms, and nearly all the muscles of the body. By the judicious use of them, a weak and sickly person can become strong and healthy. Their great advantage over dumb-bells and other implements used in calisthenics is their endless variety of exercises. They afford more scope for invention than any other kind of athletics, hence their great attraction to those who use them. There are hundreds of ways of wielding them, and every new exercise is the means of finding another.

The clubs can be used as well by children, either boys or girls, as by men and women. Clubs are particularly advantageous to ladies, who are generally prevented from doing as great an amount of exercise as men. Gymnastics proper they do not do; their calisthenics I will not mention. To them, therefore, the clubs ought to be a great boon. It is a very graceful and healthy exercise, and with all the details they will find in this book they ought to be able to become very proficient with them deriving at the same time great benefit. Of all the exercises I have given there is not one that will injure them—that is, if they practice with a club of a proper weight. This is the most important thing of all. People will use clubs too heavy for them, and thus injure themselves; it is not the exercise that hurts them, it is the weight of the club. For children from 10 to 12 years old I should advise clubs of 1lb. each, or even less should they be weak; from 12 to 15, 1½lbs., if weak only 1lb.; for boys from 15 to 17, 2lbs.; from 17 upwards, up to 4lbs., according to strength. For girls from 15 to 18, 1¾lbs.; from 18 upwards, up to 2½lbs., according to strength.

The shape of the clubs is also most important. It is very difficult to find a proper shaped club ready made; they are often turned by people who have not the slightest notion of what is done with them, and accordingly make only a clumsy round piece of wood with a handle to it, and call it a club. A club should be turned quite plain, without any ornamentation about it in the way of turning. The shape should be as shown in the following illustrations:—

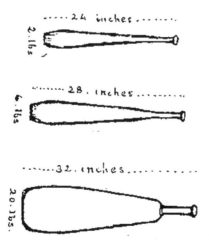

The length of a 1lb. club ought to be about 20 inches; of a 2lbs. 24 inches; and of a 4lbs., 28 inches. A heavy club should be about 32 inches long. The price of clubs is from 6d. to 9d. per lb.

In the chapter on heavy clubs will be found the necessary instructions and advice respecting the weights and use of heavy clubs. Ladies should not use heavy clubs.

Another great advantage connected with clubs is that they can be used in any room where there is a clear space of two yards by four yards, and where, of course, the ceiling is sufficiently high to allow of the clubs clearing it without touching. Those living in the suburbs, and having a little open space at the back of their house, can derive great enjoyment and benefit out of half-an-hour's quiet practice with the clubs. There is no trouble in bringing or taking them away, and they are easily put aside in a corner or out of sight.

Thus it can easily be seen that Indian Club practice affords, more than any other exercise, facilities for healthy recreation to those who from occupation or other causes are prevented from joining a gymnasium, or leading an active athletic life. To them, if they act according to all my directions, I hope the following chapters will be of great help, as such is my intention in writing this book.

I shall not give, as appears customary in books on athletics, any special notion as regards what one ought or ought not to do to preserve his or her health, how to train, when to get up, or go to bed. My object is to teach Indian Clubs to the best of my ability. I shall only say this. Above all things remember not to begin by doing much at first; five to ten minutes gentle exercise is sufficient to begin with; in fact, leave off immediately on feeling tired, and do not begin with any weight heavier than those I recommend.

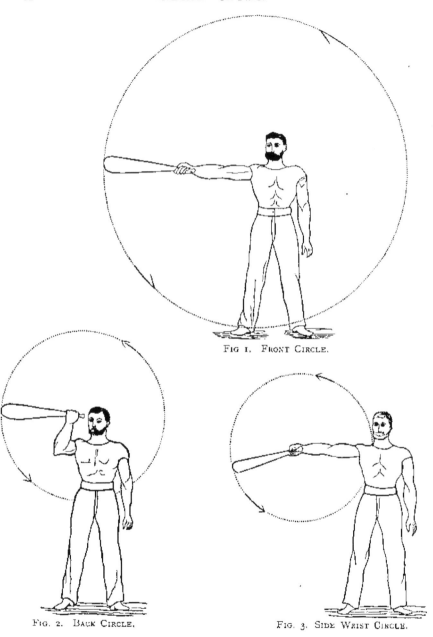

FIG 1. FRONT CIRCLE.

FIG. 2. BACK CIRCLE.

FIG. 3. SIDE WRIST CIRCLE.

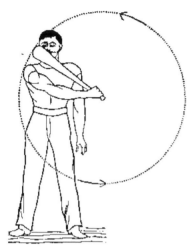

FIG. 4. FRONT WRIST CIRCLE.

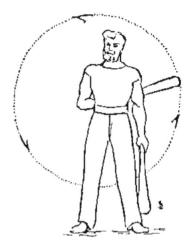

FIG. 5. LOWER BACK CIRCLE.

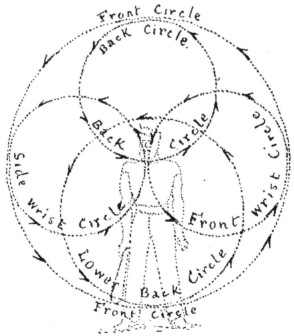

RESPECTIVE POSITION OF THE CIRCLES OF THE FIRST SERIES.

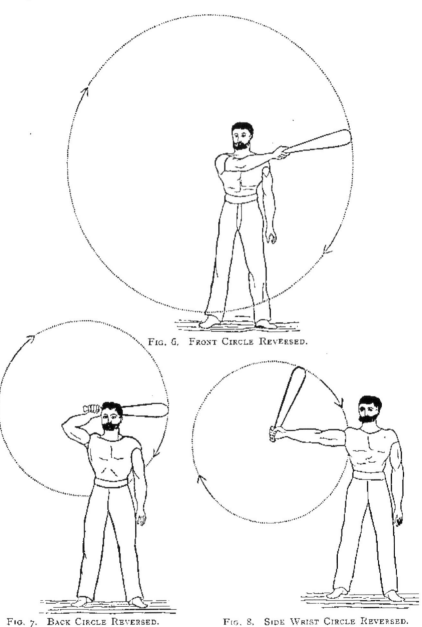

FIG. 6. FRONT CIRCLE REVERSED.

FIG. 7. BACK CIRCLE REVERSED.

FIG. 8. SIDE WRIST CIRCLE REVERSED.

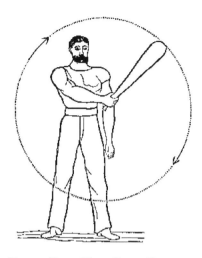

Fig. 9. Front Wrist Circle Reversed.   Fig. 10.   Lower Back Circle Reversed.

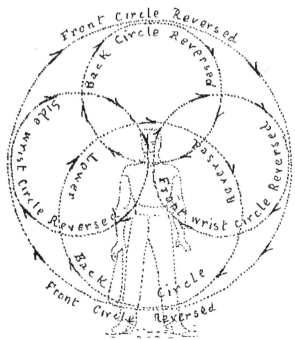

Respective Position of the Circles of the Second Series.

CHAPTER I.

PRELIMINARY REMARKS AND KEY EXERCISES.

INDIAN Club exercises are perhaps the most difficult to explain clearly and comprehensibly in a book. I have endeavoured to bring the whole to its simplest form, and for that purpose I have made a key, which will be found immediately preceding this chapter. A reference to that key will show that I have divided the exercises into three series. The whole art of the Indian Clubs is comprised in the ten figures there represented. The most intricate exercises are only a combination of those ten figures. The second series is merely the first series done backwards, and the third series is a combination of the first and the second; for this reason there are no figures in the key representing the third series. The exercises comprised in this series will be found in their proper places in the book.

It will be noticed that I have given a name to all the various circles represented in the key. It will also be seen that in the second series I have added the word "reversed"; it is to facilitate the understanding as to how the exercise should be done; for, having mastered an exercise of the first series, going from right to left, the corresponding exercise in the second series is the club travelling back in the opposite direction, or "reverse" way, from left to right. Now I want special attention to be paid to the direction of the arrows in the dotted circles which represent, in the figures, the direction the clubs are to go. The direction of the right club is marked by dotted lines thus.............. .... the direction of the left by a line of small strokes thus - - - - -

In the key all the exercises are represented as done with the right arm; and it will be seen that the exercises of the first series, when

B

done with the right arm, all go from the right to the left, passing downwards; and the exercises of the second series, done with the right arm, all go from left to right, passing downwards. But if the left arm is used instead of the right, then the exercises of the first series go from left to right, and those of the second from right to left. All this is very important to beginners, as it must greatly facilitate quick learning if thoroughly understood. It may seem very intricate in print, but if, whilst this is read, a club is held to demonstrate what I say, and is made to follow my directions, then all this will at once be understood and perhaps remembered.

I am particularly anxious to afford all the practical information that I think necessary at the beginning, as there is nothing like a good start.

Beginners should never try the more complicated exercises until they have thoroughly mastered the more simple ones. They will then be accustomed to the handling of the clubs, and be better prepared for the more difficult combinations. Do not hurry through the exercises, so as to have time to use the brain, which in the Indian Club exercises is much required, especially when both clubs are used at the same time.

I shall now explain the key, which must be first learnt, with the exception of the fifth circle of each series. These ought not to be attempted until sufficiently proficient; I shall introduce them where I think best. The various circles should be known by the names I have given them, as they will greatly help when we go further, and will save a great amount of unnecessary repetition, enabling me to refer to them simply by their names, and thus the learner will at once understand what is meant when he finds those names used in the description of the various combinations explained further in the book. I shall also adopt the same system with regard to figures. I shall first explain the figure thoroughly if need be, and afterwards the mere mention of the figure will mean that the clubs are to be used or held as represented in the said figure. I must particularly request great attention to be paid to the position of the clubs, arms and hands, as represented in the figures.

The starting position of all exercises with the Indian Clubs is shown for one arm in fig. 12, for both arms in fig. 13. Previous to getting ready for any exercise, and after doing it, the clubs can either be put down or held as in fig. 11.

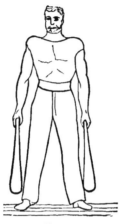

Fig. 11.

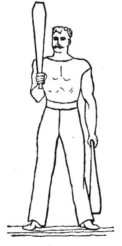

Fig. 12.

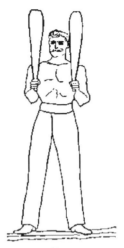

FIG. 13.

The feet should be about 18 inches apart, so as to give steadiness to the body, which ought to be erect and yet not stiff. The proper position of the feet is observed in the illustrations. Great attention must be paid to neatness and to a good position of the body, as besides giving a graceful appearance it will allow a more even play for the various muscles at work. The arms should move freely ; no ugly jerks, which are apt to

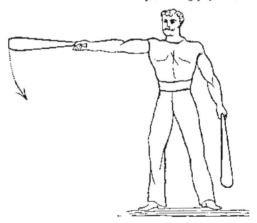

FIG. 14.

injure the elbow joint sometimes severely. In a word, the clubs ought always to be swung with grace and ease, and with a regular motion.

Do not follow the club as if attracted by its weight, as shown in figs. 14 and 15.

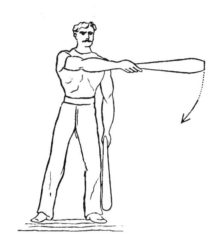

FIG. 15.

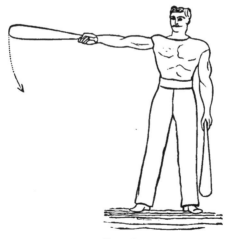

FIG. 16.

This bad habit, by shortening the distance from the shoulder to the feet, often causes the club to strike the toes.   Lean slightly in the opposite direction to that in which the club is going (figs. 16 and 17).

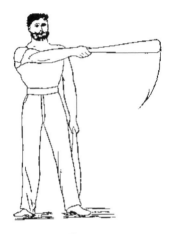

FIG. 17.

This advice will be found most useful when using rather heavy clubs, and the better it is attended to, the heavier the clubs can be.

Working before a looking-glass is of great assistance, as it helps to obtain accuracy and a good position, besides reflecting any faults that may occur.

Of course the pupil is supposed to know thoroughly one exercise before he attempts another.   If that rule is followed it will be seen how easy everything will come later on, as I have so divided the exercises and series that one works into the other.   As regards the series, I shall keep the same progression of exercises for all, so that if the order of the first series is well known, that of the second will be already known before even having begun to learn them.   However, at the end of the book will be found a table giving directions as to the order the exercises of each series should be learnt.   My reason for doing this is that thus the three series will be gradually learnt at the same time, and also it will give time to the pupil to become proficient with some of the more simple exercises of the three series before he comes to the more difficult ones.

Now to proceed with the exercises forming the key. All the exercises may be done about twelve to fifteen times in succession.

Front Circle.—Figs. 1 and 18. Take hold of the clubs as in fig. 11;

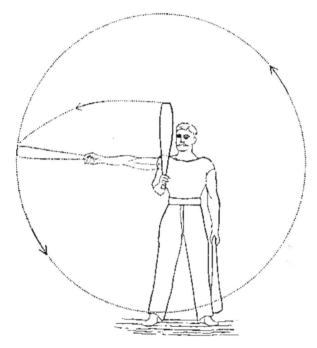

Fig. 18

then put right arm up in the starting position as in fig. 12; this starting position is also shown in fig. 18. From there thrust the club to the right, with straight arm, as shown by the dotted arm and club in fig. 18; describe a perfect circle with straight arm, passing the club in front of the body in the direction of the arrows in the dotted circles of figs. 1 and 18. Do about fifteen circles in succession, then stop by returning to the starting position of fig. 12, and from there down as in fig. 11.

Front Circle with the Left Arm.—Fig. 19. The same

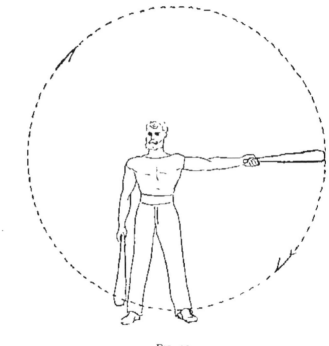

FIG. 19

exercise as the preceding, with the left arm starting of course to the left instead of the right.

Front Circle Reversed.—Figs. 6 and 20. Hold the clubs fig. 11, right arm up, fig. 12 ; from there thrust the club to the left, arm straight, as in dotted arm and club, fig. 20 ; describe a perfect circle with straight arm, passing the club in front of the body in the direction of the arrows in the dotted circles, figs. 6 and 20. Do about fifteen circles in succession, then stop by returning to the starting position, fig. 12, then down, fig. 11.

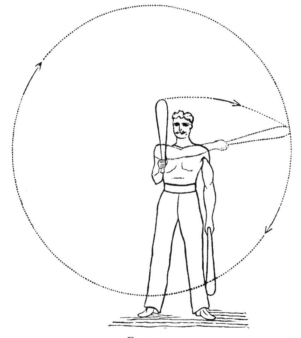

FIG. 20.

Front Circle Reversed with the Left Arm.—Same exercise as preceding with the left arm, starting the club towards the right, fig. 21.

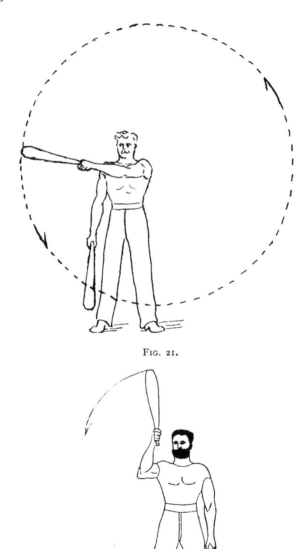

FIG. 21.

FIG. 22.

Back Circle.—Figs. 2 and 23.—Hold the club fig. 11.   Up fig. 12.
From there raise the club as in fig. 22 ; then turn it to the right as in fig.
23, holding the hand close to the right ear ; the elbow is well in front,

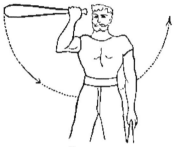

Fig. 23.

almost level with the chin, fig. 23.   Pay great attention to this position of
the elbow, as it helps much in getting this circle perfect.

From the position, fig. 23, let the club swing round behind the head in
the direction of the dotted lines, figs. 2 and 23 ; but observe that when
the club gets behind the head, as in fig. 24, the elbow changes its position
and gets quite at the side, see fig. 24 ; the club then finishes its journey
until it is again in position, fig. 22, with the elbow in front and ready to
begin another circle.

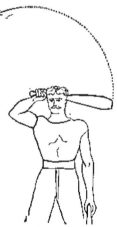

Fig. 24.

There should be no stop in this exercise, as indeed in any of the exercises with the clubs, but it is better to do this one two or three times slowly, following carefully the figures as indicated. Do the circle about fifteen times without stopping, then recover as usual, fig. 12 and fig. 11. This mode of finishing all the exercises ought now to be so well under-stood that I shall not refer to it any more. It must be made use of whenever either starting or finishing. Of course, when using both clubs at the same time, the starting and finishing is done with both clubs as shown in fig. 13. (See page 38 for remarks as to position.)

Back Circle with the Left Arm.—Same exercise as the pre-ceding, but with the left arm instead of the right, starting to the left with the end of the club well to the left. Fig. 25.

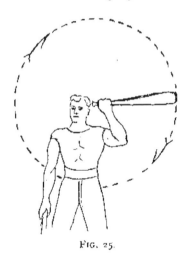

FIG. 25.

In the back circle it will be seen, by looking at the figures, that at the beginning of the circle the knuckles are facing forwards, and at the end they are facing backwards ; in fact, they follow the motion of the elbow. This action of the hand is most important.

Back Circle Reversed.—Fig. 7 and fig. 27. From the starting position raise the club as in fig. 26. Here, it must be observed, that the position of the elbow is reverse to that in the simple back circle. In the back circle reversed the elbow first gets well back, fig. 26 ; then the club

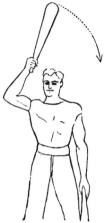

FIG. 26.

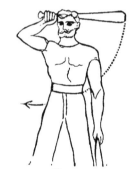

FIG. 27.

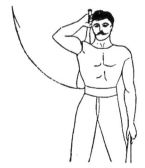

FIG. 28.

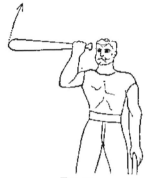

FIG. 29.

is pointed to the left and dropped behind the head in the direction of the
arrows in the dotted circles of fig. 7 and fig. 27; but when the club
arrives behind the back in the position of fig. 28, the elbow comes forward
as in fig. 29, and remains so until fig. 30.

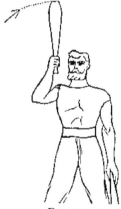

FIG. 30.

To begin another circle, resume position fig. 26, with the elbow well
back.

Do this exercise at first slowly, following the figures, and when the
exercise is well understood, do about fifteen circles in succession without
stopping. The position of the knuckles must again be observed; at the
beginning of the circle they face backwards, at the end they are forwards.

Back Circle Reversed with the Left Arm.—Same exercise as the preceding, but with the left arm instead of the right starting the club to the right, with the club pointed to the right. Fig. 31.

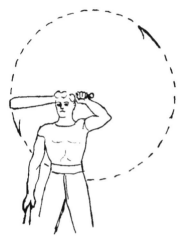

FIG. 31.

Side Wrist Circle.—Fig. 3 and fig. 32. Hold the club up with the right arm, as shown in fig. 33.

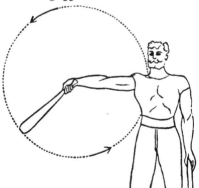

FIG. 32.

The arm is straight. Swing the club, by dropping it away from the body, in the direction of the arrows in the dotted lines, describing a circle, the

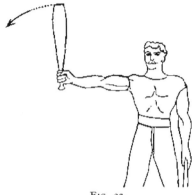

FIG. 33.

club passing behind the arm, as in figure 34. When the club starts, the
nails of the fingers are upwards, as shown in fig. 35; and when it has
almost completed the circle, the nails are downwards, as in fig. 36.   To

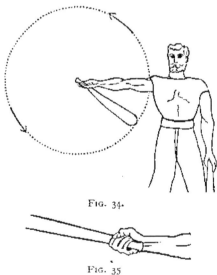

FIG. 34.

FIG. 35

begin another circle, sharply turn the wrist, so that the nails again face
upwards. Fig. 35.

The whole science of the wrist circle is contained in that turning of
the wrist.

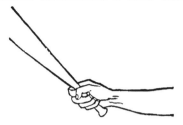

FIG. 36.

Side Wrist Circle with the Left Arm.—Proceed with the left arm in the same manner as explained in the preceding exercise. Fig. 37.

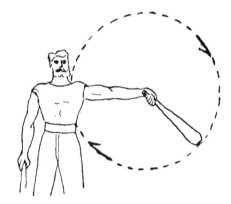

FIG. 37.

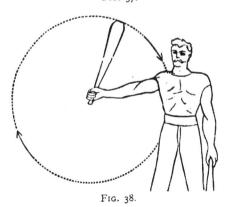

FIG. 38.

D

Side Wrist Circle Reversed.—Figs. 8 and 38. Hold the club up with the right arm, as in fig. 33. Swing the club by dropping it towards the body, the club passing behind the arm—fig. 39—and in the direction of the arrows in the dotted circles, figs. 38 and 39, describing a circle.

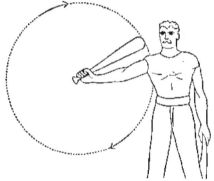

FIG. 39.

Fig. 40 shows the position of the hand at starting, and fig. 41 the position at the finish of the circle.

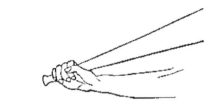

FIG. 40.

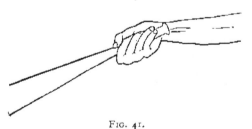

FIG. 41.

Side Wrist Circle Reversed with the Left Arm.—The same as the preceding, but with the left arm instead of the right. Fig. 42.

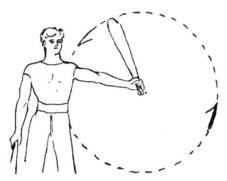

Fig. 42.

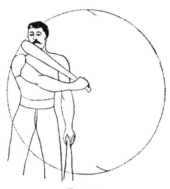

Fig. 43.

Front Wrist Circle.—Figs. 4 and 43. Hold the club up with the right arm as shown in fig. 44; the arm is straight. Swing the club by dropping it towards the right shoulder in the direction of the arrows in the dotted circle of fig. 43, and passing the club behind the arm as shown in fig. 45. The position of the hands in this exercise is exactly the same as in the side wrist circle reversed, figs. 40 and 41.

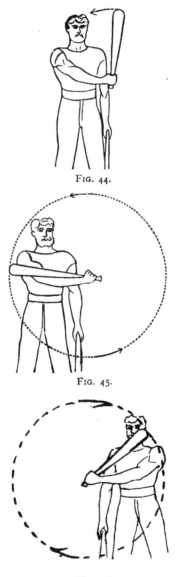

FIG. 44.

FIG. 45.

FIG. 46.

Front Wrist Circle with the Left Arm.—The same as the preceding, but with the left arm instead of the right. Fig. 46.

Front Wrist Circle Reversed.—Figs. 9 and 47. Hold the club

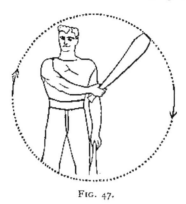

FIG. 47.

up with the right arm as shown in fig. 44 Swing the club by dropping it outwards, away from the body, in the direction of the arrows in the dotted circle of fig. 47, and passing the club behind the arm as shown in

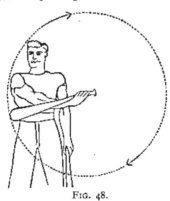

FIG. 48.

fig. 48. The position of the hands in this exercise is exactly the same as in the side wrist circle, figs 35 and 36.

Front Wrist Circle Reversed with the Left Arm.—Same as the preceding, but with the left arm instead of the right. Fig. 49.

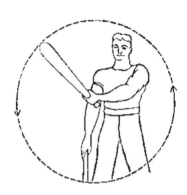

FIG. 49.

Important.—In all the wrist circles the arm does not move from its position ; the wrist alone must be used.

The pupil has now gone through eight of the exercises, or circles denominated in the key, Nos. 5 and 10 having been purposely left out until the pupil is sufficiently advanced for them to be of some use to him. These will be introduced in their proper place.

It is absolutely necessary that the first eight exercises above mentioned should be thoroughly learnt before anything further is attempted, for when they are quite mastered the remainder will come with comparative ease, the whole of the exercises with the Indian Clubs being, as I have already stated, merely a combination of the circles appearing in the key.

At the beginning of this chapter I have pointed out the bad habit to avoid in doing the front circle. I shall now mention what is right and what is wrong in doing the back circle.

1st.—In all the back circles the right hand must remain near the right ear, and the left hand near the left ear, figs. 50 and 51. Not only is this the right position, but it will save many blows on the head, for if the hand is away from the ear, the result often is as shown in fig. 52, which cannot possibly happen if the hand is in its proper place.

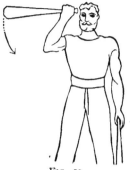

FIG. 50.

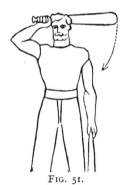

FIG. 51.

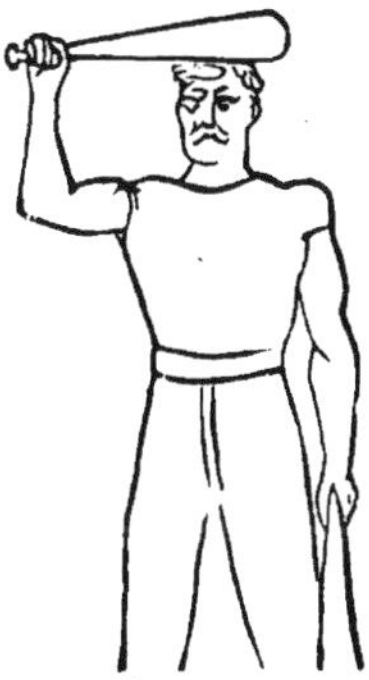

FIG. 52.

2nd.—In all back circles the elbow must be well up, as in figs. 50 and 51, and not as in figs. 53 and 54.

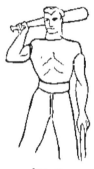

FIG 53.

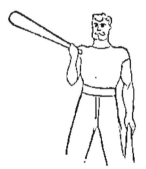

FIG. 54.

3rd.—Do not bend the knees or lean the head on one side when doing a back circle, as is shown in figs. 55 and 56. Many do it thinking they thus avoid a blow on the head, or help to jerk the club off. Keep perfectly erect, as in figs. 2 and 7.

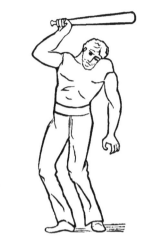

FIG. 55.

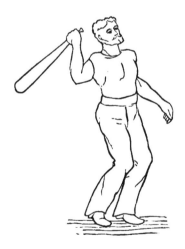

FIG. 56.

I think I have given in this chapter nearly all the practical information and hints which experience has taught me, and I hope they will be fully appreciated. I have no doubt that if well kept in mind they will prove of the greatest advantage to the beginner ; and for this reason I recommend him to read over this chapter occasionally, even when he is learning the most complicated exercises, as it will refresh his memory should he have forgotten any of my instructions.

CHAPTER II.

I SHALL now proceed with the first series of exercises. Every exercise will be numbered for further reference. I shall also give "counting time" to all exercises. The numbers appearing by the side of the dotted circles in the figures will refer to the counting which must be done when the club arrives at the place where the numbers appear. The time of counting not to be quicker than "common time" in music.

I shall not repeat any of the instructions I have given in the preceding chapter respecting position, &c., as I suppose that by this time they are well known. Do not forget about the starting positions, figs. 11, 12, and 13.

When the arm is doing a front circle it should be kept well straight. Each exercise to be done about fifteen times, counting the whole time. In no exercise must there be a stoppage in the motion of the clubs, but keep on swinging them, at the same time counting as indicated ; for example, where there are two to be counted, count *one—two, one—two, one—two,* and so on until the exercise is finished.

In the figures, the direction taken by the right club will be marked by small dots, and that of the left club by small strokes. The starting position is shown by the arms and clubs that are fully drawn. The dotted arms and clubs are to show the various positions assumed during the exercises.

First Series.

In this series the right club always goes towards the right, and the left club towards the left.

Exercise 1.—Front circle with the right arm. Count—*one*—as the club goes round. This is a key exercise and needs no further description.

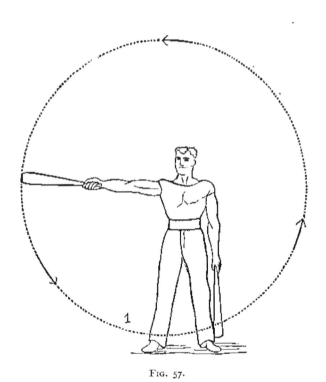

FIG. 57.

Fig. 57 shows the exercise.

Exercise 2.—Front circle with the left arm. Count—*one* – as before. Fig. 58.

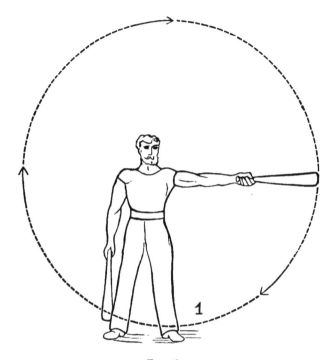

FIG. 5S.

Exercise 3.—Front circle with both arms at the same time. Fig. 59. Right club goes to the right, and left to the left. The clubs cross one another when passing the knees and above the head. See the dotted clubs in fig. 59. Count—*one*—when crossing by the knees.

Exercise 4.—Front circle with each arm alternately. Both clubs in the starting position. Throw the right arm first to the right, as in fig. 60, counting—*one*. When the right club passes the legs, throw the left club to the left (fig. 61) and count—*two*. The clubs cross one another at the side as shown in fig. 62.

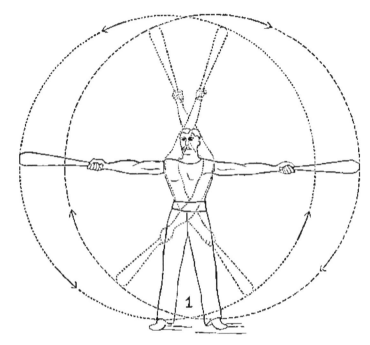

FIG. 59.

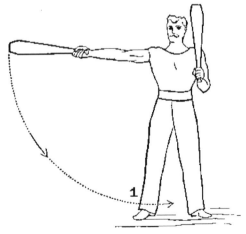

FIG. 60.

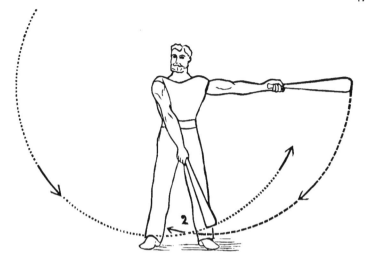

FIG. 61.

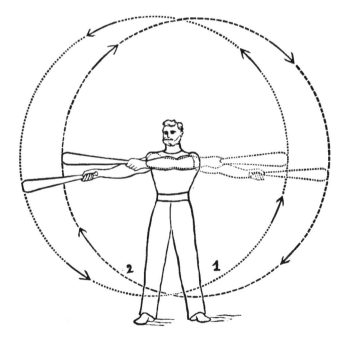

FIG. 62.

Exercise 5.—Front circle and back circle combined, with the right arm.   Throw the club to the right, doing a front circle, counting—*one.* When the front circle is completed bend the arm as in fig. 22, and do a back circle, figs. 23 and 24, counting—*two.* Then, when the circle is

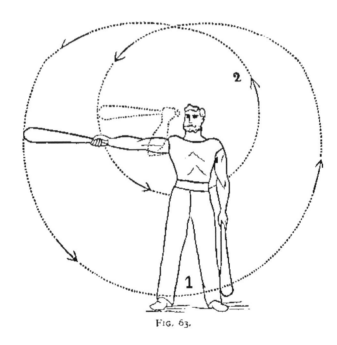

FIG. 63.

completed and the club has returned to position, fig. 22, throw the club again with straight arm to begin another front circle. This exercise is shown in fig. 63. I have fully explained in the key exercises how to do a back circle.

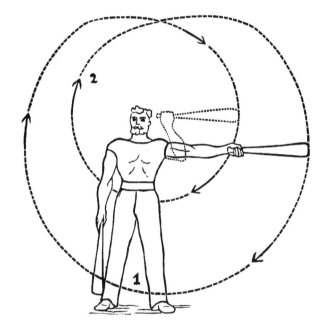

FIG. 64.

Exercise 6.—Front circle and back circle combined with the left
arm. Same as Exercise 5, but with the left arm. Throw left club to the
left, doing front circle—*one;* back circle—*two.* Fig. 64.

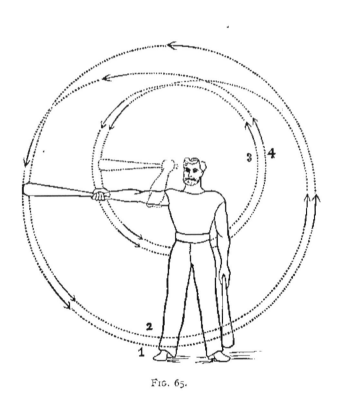

Fig. 65.

Exercise 7.—Double the Exercise 5 with the right arm by doing two front circles in succession—*one—two*, and two back circles—*three— four*. Fig. 65.

Exercise 8.—The same as Exercise 7 with the left arm.

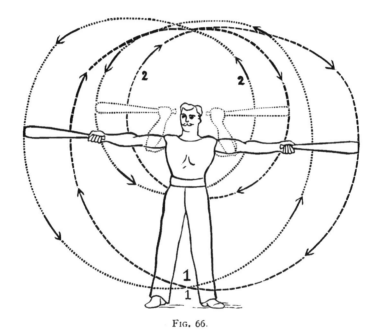

FIG. 66.

Exercise 9.—Front circle and back circle with both arms at the
same time.   Describe a front circle with both arms as in Exercise 3,
count—*one;* and then do a back circle with both arms, count—*two.*
Fig. 66.   E 2

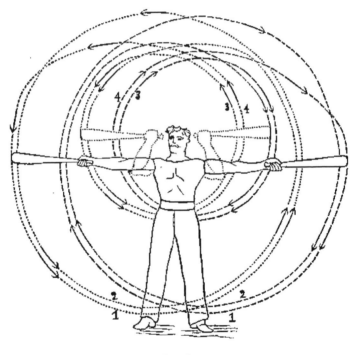

F<small>IG</small>. 67

Exercise 10.—Double Exercise 9, by doing two front circles with both arms—*one—two*, and two back circles with both arms—*three—four*. Fig. 67.

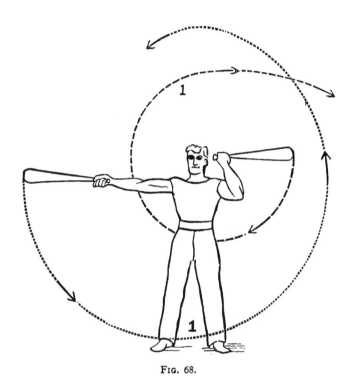

FIG. 68.

Exercise 11.—Front circle with one arm and back circle with the other at the same time. Though both arms are working simultaneously the circles of the same category are done alternately. Both clubs start at the same time. The right club starts to do a front circle and the left club to do a back circle, counting—*one*. This first start and circles are shown in fig. 68.

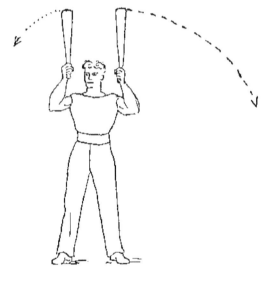

FIG. 69.

When the right club has finished the front circle, the left club has also finished the back circle, both clubs being then in position (fig. 69), that is to say, the starting position (the clubs, however, are held higher

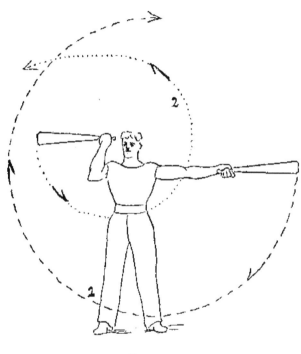

F<small>IG.</small> 70

than in the ordinary starting position, fig. 13); from there the right club
this time does a back circle and the left club a front circle, both at the
same time, counting—*two*. This is shown in fig. 70.

When the circles are completed, the clubs are again in the starting position, fig. 69; then begin again, right club in front, left back—*one*, left club front and right club back—*two*, and so on alternately.   Fig. 71 shows the whole exercise.

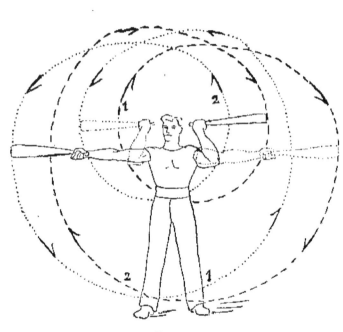

FIG. 71.

Of course, when the way the clubs are to go is well understood, there should be no stoppage noticeable at the position, fig. 69.   Both clubs then are kept in motion.   It will be noticed that this exercise is simply Exercise 5 done alternately with each arm, one arm having started "*one time*" behind the other.

Exercise 12.—Double Exercise 11 with each arm. Start exactly as in Exercise 11, but, instead of one circle with each arm, do two front circles with the right while the left does two back circles. Time, after first circle—*one*, second circle—*two*. When the second set of circles is

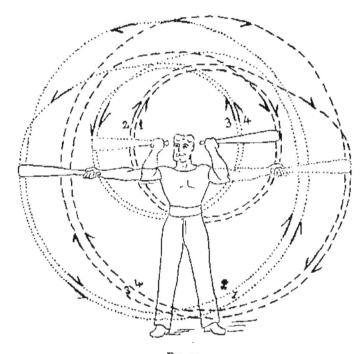

FIG. 72.

completed, do two front circles with the left, doing at the same time two back circles with the right, counting—*three—four* (fig. 72). This Exercise is the same as Exercise 7, done alternately with each arm.

Exercise 13.—A combination of Exercises 3 and 11. First do a front circle with both arms at the same time, fig. 59, count—*one;* then a front circle with the right arm and back circle with the left, fig. 68, count —*two;* then do again a front circle with both arms, fig. 59—*three;* and after that a front circle with the left arm and back circle with the right, fig. 70—*four.* The whole exercise is shown by fig. 73.

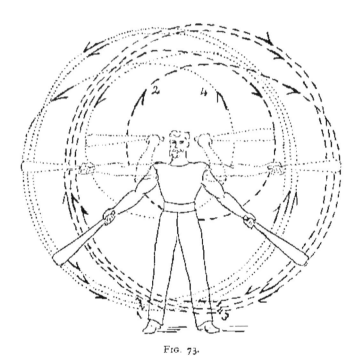

FIG. 73.

Exercise 14.—Double the preceding by doing two front circles with both arms at the same time—*one—two;* then, as in Exercise 12, two front circles with the right whilst the left does two back circles—*three— four,* as in fig. 72; then again two front circles with both arms at the same time—*five—six;* after which two front circles with the left whilst the right does two back circles—*seven—eight.*

Exercise 15.—Side wrist circle with the right club, fig. 74. Count —*one*—as the club goes round. This being a key exercise it needs no description.

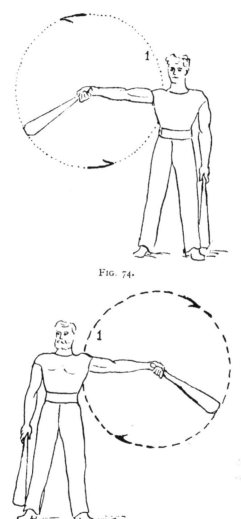

FIG. 74.

FIG. 75.

Exercise 16.—Side wrist circle with the left club, fig. 75—*one*.

Exercise 17.—A combination of exercises 5 and 15 with the right club. That is, front circle—*one*, then back circle—*two*, then side wrist circle—*three*. Start as in Exercise 5; do that exercise completely in the manner already described, fig. 63. When, after the back circle, the arm is thrown out straight to begin another front circle, as shown in fig. 63, before doing that front circle do a side wrist circle, after which then do a front circle, then a back, then a side wrist and so on, counting—*one—two—three*. This exercise is shown in fig. 76.

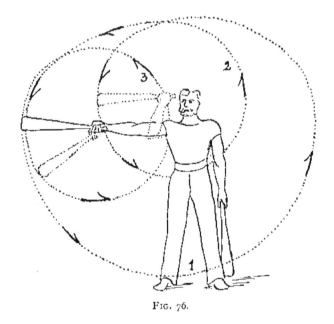

FIG. 76.

Exercise 18.—The same exercise with the left; a combination of Exercises 6 and 16. Front circle—*one*, back circle—*two*, side wrist circle—*three*.

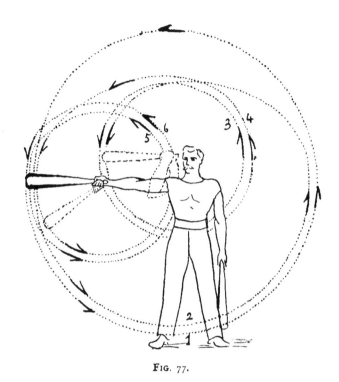

FIG. 77.

Exercise 19.—Double Exercise 17 with the right arm. What I mean by doubling ought now to be easily understood, so this exercise will need hardly any detailing. Do two consecutive front circles—*one—two;* two consecutive back circles—*three—four;* two consecutive side wrist circles—*five—six.* This exercise is shown in fig. 77.

Exercise 20.—Same exercise as the preceding with the left club.

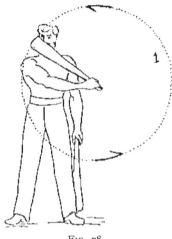

FIG. 78.

Exercise 21.—Front wrist circle with the right club. Fig. 78.
This, being another key exercise, needs no further description.   Count
—*one*.

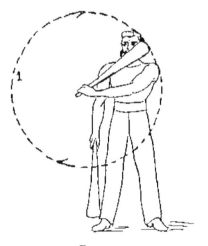

FIG. 79.

Exercise 22.—Front wrist circle with the left club. Fig. 79.

Exercise 23.—A combination of Exercises 5 and 21. In this exercise the front circle and the back circle of Exercise 5 are divided by the front wrist circle. First start, as in Exercise 5, to do a front circle, counting—*one.* When the club has described half the circle, and the arm is in front of the body, as in fig. 78, do a front wrist circle,

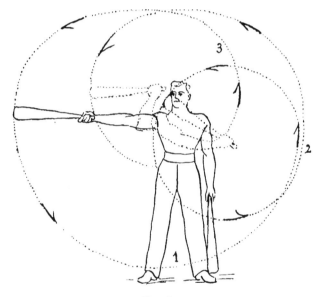

Fig. 80.

counting—*two.* When this is done, finish the front circle by letting the club go upwards, then do a back circle—*three.* Begin again as before with front circle. Fig. 80 shows the whole exercise.

Exercise 24.—The same as the preceding, with the left arm. Part of front circle—*one ;* front wrist circle—*two ;* back circle—*three.* Fig. 81.

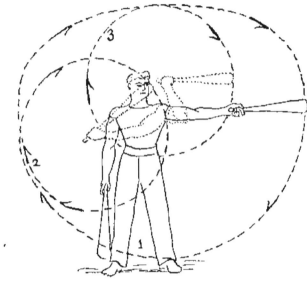

FIG. 81.

Exercise 25.—Double Exercise 23 with the right arm.   First one complete front circle—*one ;* then part of another until the club gets in front, as in fig. 78—*two ;* then two successive front wrist circles—*three—four ;* then two successive back circles—*five—six.*

Exercise 26.—Same as the preceding, with the left arm.

Exercise 27.—A combination of Exercises 17 and 23, or perhaps, more correctly, Exercise 23, to which is added the side wrist circle after the back circle.

Do the whole of Exercise 23 as already detailed, that is, part of the front circle—*one ;* front wrist circle—*two ;* back circle—*three ;* but when the back circle is completed proceed as in Exercise 17, that is, throw the arm out straight as if to begin another front circle, but before doing that front circle describe a side wrist circle, and count—*four ;* when this is done begin again by letting the club go downwards, doing part of a front circle, counting—*one ;* then a front wrist circle—*two ;* then back circle—*three ;* then side wrist circle—*four;* and so on. This exercise is shown in fig. 82.

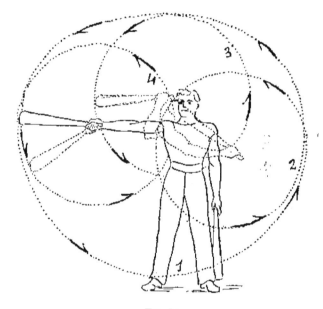

Fig. 82.

It will be seen by following the lines that, no matter what the circle is, the club always goes in the same direction. Here we have four circles and yet the club does not once change its way of going. F

Exercise 28.—The same exercise as 27 with the left club; same counting. Fig. 83.

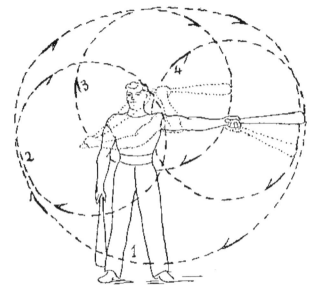

FIG. 83.

Exercise 29.—Double Exercise 27 with the right arm.   One complete front circle—*one;* part of front circle—*two;* two successive front wrist circles—*three—four;* two successive back circles—*five—six;* two side wrist circles—*seven—eight.*

Exercise 30.—Same as the preceding, with the left club.

Exercise 31.—A combination of Exercises 15 and 21, that is, side wrist circle with the right club and front wrist circle with the left.   Hold the clubs out, exactly as shown in fig. 84, then do a side wrist circle with the right club, doing *at the same time* a front wrist circle with the left ; count—*one.* Do this several times in succession. There must be no scrambling through the exercise, and at the first attempt it is better to stop after every set of circles, in the position fig. 84, but when perfect the stop should not be noticeable.

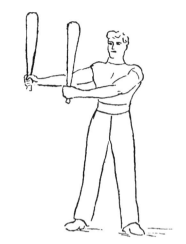

FIG 84.

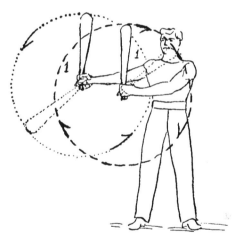

FIG. 85.

The exercise is shown in fig. 85. I need hardly say that one club goes in a contrary direction to the other, as will be seen by reference to the dotted lines.

F2

Exercise 32.—Same kind of exercise as the preceding, but this time it is the left club that does the side wrist circle, and the right club does *at the same time* a front wrist circle. The clubs are held on the left side, fig. 86. Count—*one.*

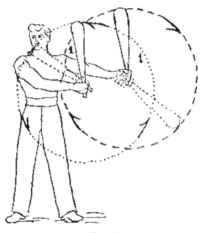

FIG. 86.

Exercise 33.—Combination of Exercises 11, 31 and 32. This is also a combination of Exercises 27 and 28.

This exercise may appear difficult and complicated to a beginner, but to the pupil who has arrived at this stage gradually, by following the order I have set down, it ought to be very easy of execution. Of course the pupil is supposed to know thoroughly Exercise 11, figs. 68, 69, 70, 71. This Exercise 33 is Exercise 32 done after the first half of Exercise 11, and Exercise 31 done after the second half of Exercise 11.

Start as shown fig. 68; front circle with the right club, at the same time back circle with the left club, count—*one;* when this is done the clubs in the ordinary way ought to be in position fig. 69, but in the present exercise they should be held a little to the left as in fig. 87; then straighten the arms to the left as shown in fig. 86, doing almost at the same time Exercise 32, count—*two;* after which resume position fig. 87. Then do a front circle with the left arm, at the same time back circle with the right, fig. 70, count—*three.* After this the position is as shown in fig. 88, that

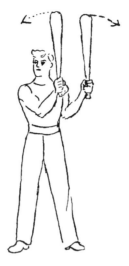

FIG. 87.

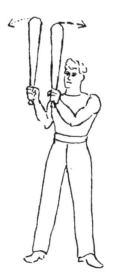

FIG. 88.

is, the clubs held a little to the right; now straighten the arms to the right as in fig. 85, doing at the same time Exercise 31—count—*four;* resume position of fig. 88 and begin the exercise again. Time—*one—two— three—four.*

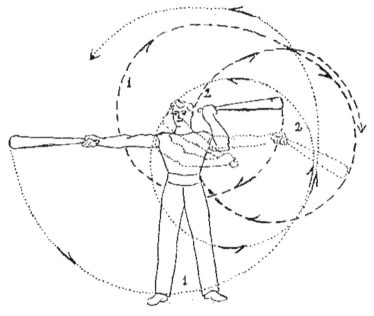

Fig. 89.

This exercise is shown, for times—*one—two*—in fig. 89; for times— *three—four*—in fig. 90; and the whole of the exercise in fig. 91.

Exercise 34.—The pupil may now try to double the exercise by doing two consecutive circles of each class—right club two front circles, left club two back circles—*one—two;* right club two front wrist circles, left club two side wrist circles—*three—four;* right club two back circles, left club two front circles—*five—six;* right club two side wrist circles and left club two front wrist circles—*seven—eight.*

Exercise 35.—A combination of Exercises 3 and 33, figs. 59 and 91. This exercise is simply Exercise 33, to which is added a front circle with both arms, that is Exercise 3, after each half of the exercise, or otherwise after fig. 89 and after fig. 90.

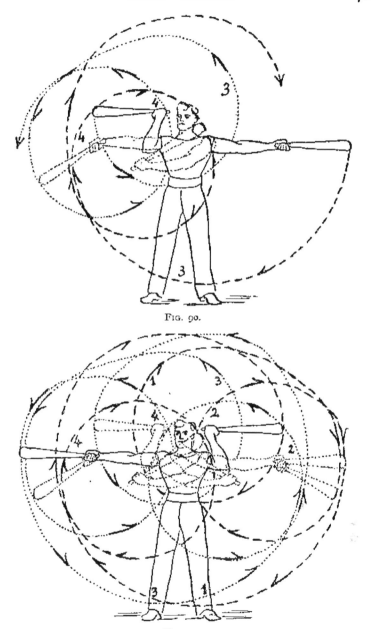

FIG. 90.

FIG. 91.

It is also a combination of Exercises 13, 31 and 32, figs. 73, 85 and 86.

Begin exactly as in Exercise 13; but after time—*two*—do Exercise 32, fig. 86; then again as in Exercise 13, and after time—*four*—of that exercise, do Exercise 31, fig. 85. The counting is—*one—two—three—four—five—six.*

Exercise 36.—Front circle and front wrist circle combined with each club alternately.

Begin by a front circle with the right club and at the same time do a front wrist circle with the left, counting—*one;* fig. 92. The right arm

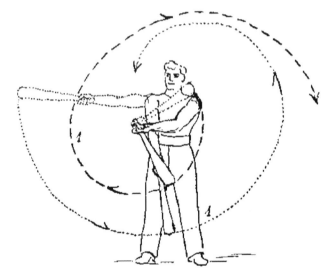

FIG. 92

passes between the body and the left club, as represented in fig. 92. The dotted clubs in the figure show the position of the clubs just after starting. The right arm, instead of being perfectly straight when finishing the front circle, bends a little, so as to get more easily into the position for the front wrist circle. The left club, after doing the front wrist circle, is thrown with straight arm to the left to do a front circle, the right club doing at the same time a front wrist circle, fig. 93, count—*two.* The dotted circles in fig. 93 begin where those of fig. 92 finish, so that by looking at both figures the whole course of the clubs during the exercise can be followed.

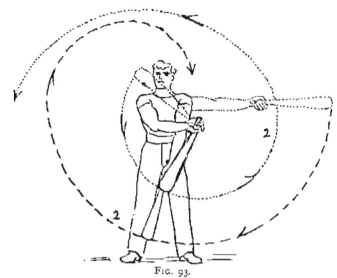

FIG. 93.

Exercise 37.—A combination of Exercises 36, 31 and 32. Start as in the previous exercise, but after time—*one*—fig. 92, do Exercise 32, fig. 86, after which, as in Exercise 36, front circle with the left club, at the same time front wrist circle with the right, fig. 93, then Exercise 31, fig. 85. Time—*one—two—three—four.* Fig. 94 shows this exercise.

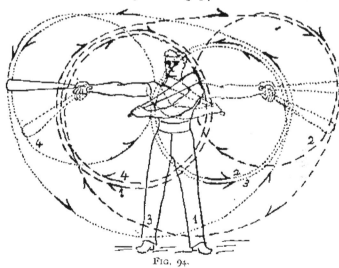

FIG. 94.

Exercise 38.—Double Exercise 37; that is, double every circle. The pupil must now be so far advanced that there is no need to detail this exercise at length. The time is—*one—two—three—four—five—six—seven—eight.*

Exercise 39.—Front circle with one club, doing at the same time a back circle and a side wrist circle with the other. This exercise is the same as Exercise 11, to which is added a side wrist circle done by the club that has completed a back circle. Begin as in Exercise 11, but the right club must do the front circle in a slower time, so that whilst it is doing that front circle, the left club has time to do a back circle and a side wrist circle, and for the same reason the left club must do the back circle and the side wrist circle rather sharply, so that the side wrist circle is completed at the same time as the other club finishes the front circle. Begin front circle with right club, doing at the same time with the other club a back circle, count—*one*; then straighten the left arm, and do a side wrist circle, count—*two*. Fig. 95. After that, front circle with left club,

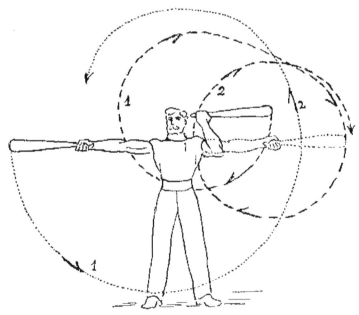

FIG. 95.

doing at same time back circle—*three*—and side wrist circle—*four*—with the right club. Fig. 96. The whole exercise is shown in fig. 97.

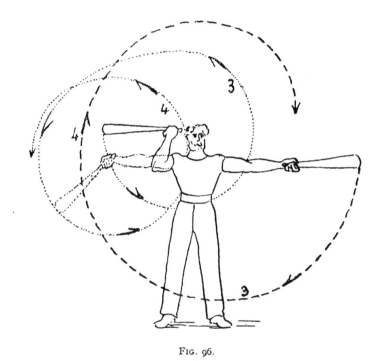

FIG. 96.

Exercise 40.—Front circle with one club, doing at the same time with the other club, firstly a front wrist circle, secondly a back circle. The directions as to the time are exactly the same as in the preceding exercise.

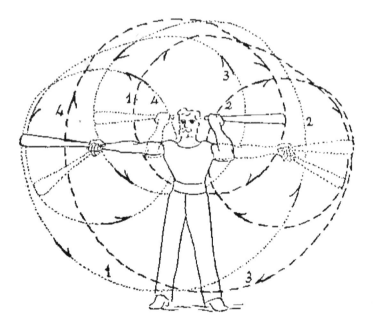

FIG. 97

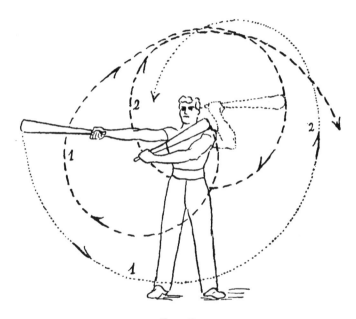

FIG. 98.

Begin front circle with right club, doing at the same time with the left, first a front wrist circle—*one*; then a back circle—*two*. Fig. 98. Then

do a front circle with the left club, and at the same time with the right,
first a front wrist circle—*three*; after which a back circle—*four*.   Fig. 99.

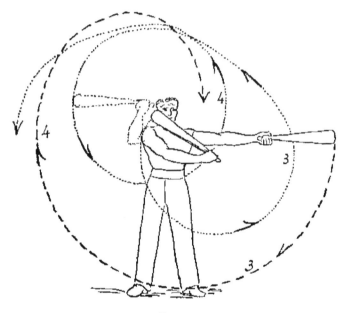

FIG. 99.

Now we have gone through most of the exercises belonging to the 1st
series.   We have done so gradually, adding one thing to another, until
even what appeared the most difficult must have really been easy to
accomplish.   I again wish to call particular attention to the fact that in

these 40 exercises the club never once changes its course whatever may be the circle. This will be seen by referring to fig. 100, as well as to all the other figures relating to the first 40 exercises.

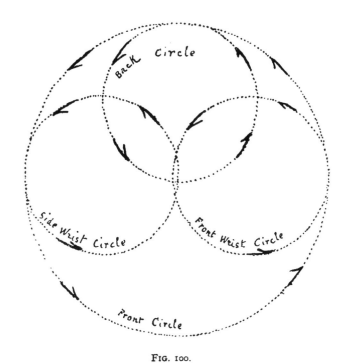

FIG. 100.

The remaining **exercises** belonging to this series will be given further on for reasons already stated.

SECOND SERIES.

Here the pupil must bear well in mind that the exercises of this series are done exactly *in the opposite direction* to those of the first series. Referring to the corresponding exercises in the first series will greatly assist in knowing how those of the second are to go. In this series the right club always goes towards the left, and the left club towards the right.

Those who have thoroughly learnt the key exercises as well as the first series will find by what I have just said that, in reality, they already know the exercises of the second series, these being only the first series reversed.

Exercise 41.—Front circle reversed with the right club, fig. 101. Count—*one.* This is a key exercise.

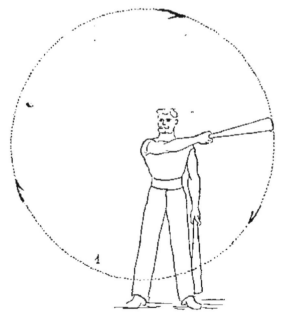

FIG. 101.

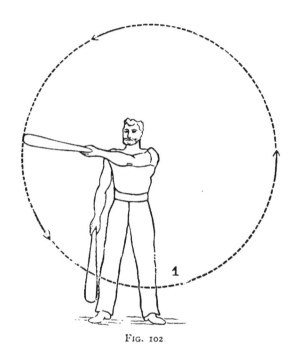

FIG. 102

Exercise 42.—Front circle reversed with the left club—*one.*
Fig. 102.

Exercise 43.—Front circle reversed with both arms. The right arm goes to the left, and the left to the right. The clubs cross one another when passing the knees and above the head (see dotted clubs). Fig. 103. Count—*one*—when crossing by the knees.

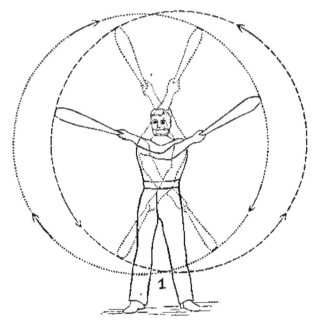

FIG. 103.

Exercise 44.—Front circle reversed with each arm alternately. Hold both clubs in the starting position. Throw the right club first to the left. Fig. 104—*one*. When the right club passes the legs throw the left club to the right. Fig. 105—*two*. The clubs cross one another at the side as in fig. 62.

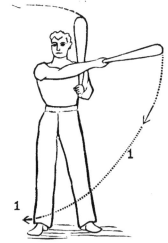

FIG. 104.

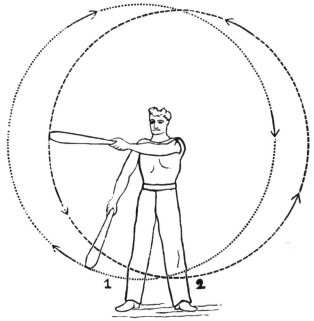

FIG. 105.

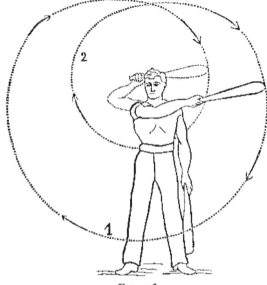

FIG. 106.

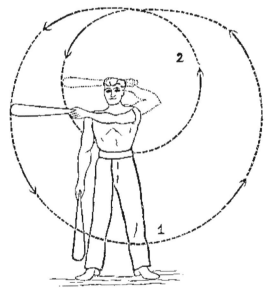

FIG. 107.

Exercise 45.—Front circle reversed and back circle reversed with the right club. Throw the club to the left, doing a front circle reversed—*one*. When this is done bend the arm as in Fig. 26, and do a back circle reversed (figs. 27, 28, 29, 30)—*two*. After this throw the club again with straight arm to the left, to begin another front circle reversed. This exercise is shown in fig. 106. The way to do a back circle reversed has been fully explained in the key exercises.

Exercise 46.—Same as Exercise 45, but with the left club. Throw left club to the right; front circle reversed—*one*; back circle reversed—*two*. Fig. 107.

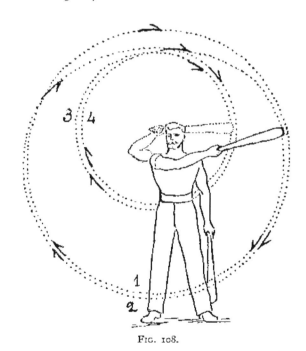

FIG. 108.

Exercise 47.—Double Exercise 45, with the right club, by doing two front circles reversed, in succession—*one—two*, and two back circles reversed, in succession—*three—four*. Fig. 108.

Exercise 48.—The same as Exercise 47, with the left club—*one—two—three—four,*

Exercise 49.—Front circle reversed and back circle reversed with both arms at the same time.

Do a front circle reversed with both arms as Exercise˜43, fig. 103—*one*; after which, back circle reversed, with both arms at the same time—*two.* Fig. 109.

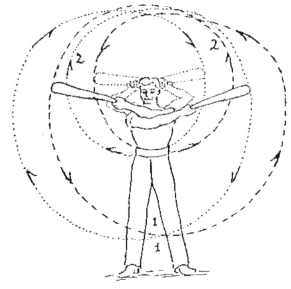

Fɪɢ. 109.

Exercise 50.—Double Exercise 49. Two consecutive front circles reversed with both arms *at the same time—one—two*; and two consecutive back circles reversed with both arms at the same time—*three—four.*

Exercise 51.—Front circle reversed with one arm, and back circle reversed with the other at the the same time.

Though both arms are working simultaneously, the circles of the same category are done alternately. Both clubs start at the same time; the right club starts to do a front circle reversed, and the left club a back circle reversed, counting *one.* The first start and circles are shown in fig. 110. When the right club has finished the front circle reversed,

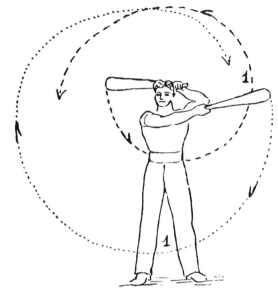

FIG. 110.

the left club *must* also have finished the back circle reversed, both clubs being then in position (fig. 111)—that is to say, the starting

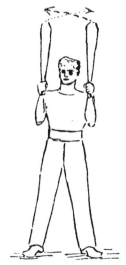

FIG. 111.

position. (The clubs, however, are held higher than in the ordinary starting position, fig. 13). From there the right club this time does a back circle reversed, and the left club a front circle reversed, both at the same time, counting *two*. Fig. 112. When the circles are com-

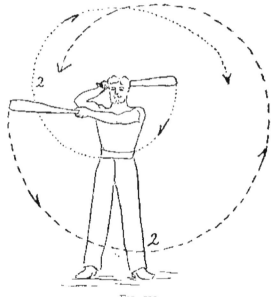

Fig. 112.

pleted the clubs are again in the starting position (fig. 111), and then begin again, right club in front, left club back—*one*; left club front, right club back—*two*, and so on alternately. The whole exercise is shown in fig. 113.

When the exercise is well understood there should be no stoppage noticeable at position fig. 111. Both clubs should be kept going.

This exercise is Exercise 45 done alternately with each arm, both arms working at the same time.

Exercise 52.—Double Exercise 51. This needs no detailing. It is also the same as Exercise 47 done alternately with each arm. Fig. 114. Time—*one—two—three—four*.

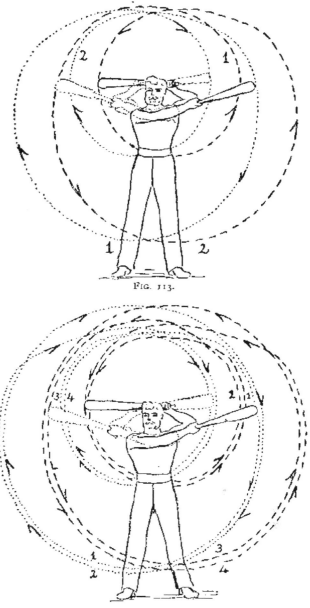

FIG. 113.

FIG. 114.

Exercise 53.—A combination of Exercise 43 and Exercise 51. First do a front circle reversed with both arms *at the same time* (fig. 103) —*one*; then a front circle reversed with the right club and a back circle reversed *at the same time* with the left (fig. 110)—*two*; after that do again a front circle reversed with both arms (fig. 103)—*three*; and then a front circle reversed with the left club and a back circle reversed with the right (fig. 112)—*four*. The whole exercise is shown in fig. 115.

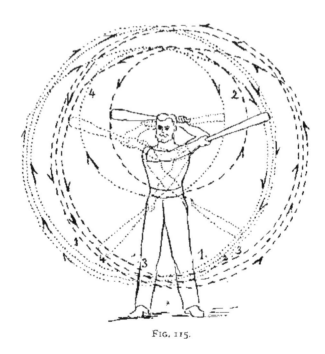

FIG. 115.

Exercise 54.—Double Exercise 53. This ought to be easily understood. Proceed in the same manner as detailed in exercise 14, but doing, of course, reversed circles instead of ordinary ones. Time—*one to eight*.

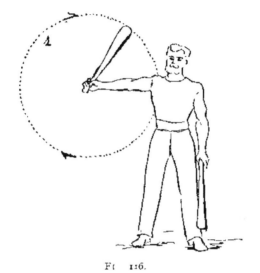

Fɩ   116.

Exercise 55.—Side wrist circle reversed with the right club. Fig. 116. Count *one* as the club goes round. This is a key exercise, and needs no description here.

Exercise 56.—Side wrist circle reversed with the left club—*one*.

Exercise 57.—A combination of Exercise 45 and Exercise 55 with the right club. Front circle reversed—*one*. Side wrist circle reversed —*two*. Back circle reversed—*three*. Start, as in Exercise 45, by doing a front circle reversed, but when the club arrives at the side, as in the position shown in fig. 116, then do a side wrist circle reversed, after which continue the front circle reversed upwards, and do a back circle reversed. This exercise is shown in fig. 117.

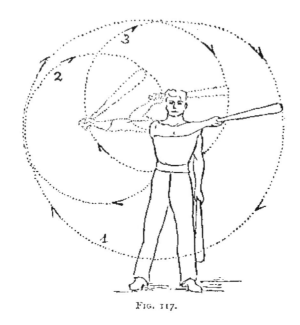

Fig. 117.

Exercise 58.—The same as Exercise 57, with the left club.

Exercise 59.—Double Exercise 57 with the right club; that is, two consecutive front circles reversed—*one—two* ; two consecutive side wrist circles reversed—*three—four*; two consecutive back circles reversed —*five—six*. Fig. 118.

Exercise 60.—Same as Exercise 59 with the left club.

Exercise 61.—Front wrist circle reversed with the right club. Fig. 119. This is a key exercise, and needs no description here.

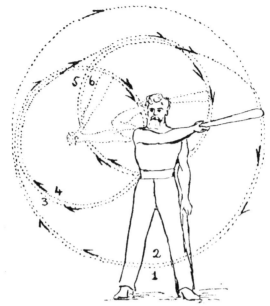

FIG. 118.

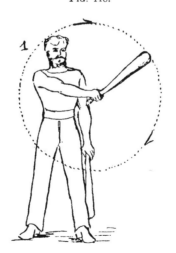

FIG. 119.

Exercise 62.—Front wrist circle reversed with the left club.

Exercise 63.—A combination of Exercise 45 and Exercise 61 with the right club. Front circle reversed—*one*; back circle reversed—*two*; front wrist circle reversed—*three.* Proceed exactly as in Exercise 45, but after doing the back circle reversed, when the arm straightens to begin another front circle reversed and gets into the position of fig. 119, do a front wrist circle reversed, after which continue the front circle reversed downwards. This exercise is shown in fig. 120.

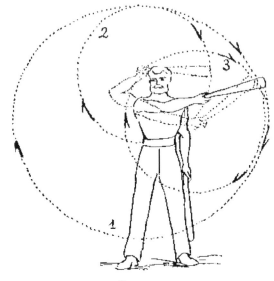

Fig. 120.

Exercise 64.—Same as Exercise 63 with the left club—*one—two —three.*

Exercise 65.—Double Exercise 63 with the right club. Two successive front circles reversed—*one—two*; two successive back circles reversed—*three—four*; two successive front wrist circles reversed—*five —six.*

Exercise 66.—Same as Exercise 65, with left club.

Exercise 67.—A combination of Exercise 55 and Exercise 63; also of Exercise 57 and Exercise 63. It is Exercise 63 to which is added the side wrist circle reversed after the front wrist circle reversed. It is also Exercise 57 to which is added a front wrist circle reversed after the back circle reversed.

Begin front circle reversed—*one* ; side wrist circle reversed—*two* ; back circle reversed—*three* ; front wrist circle reversed—*four*. Fig. 121.

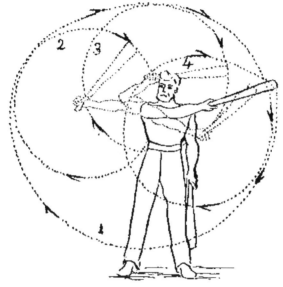

FIG. 121.

Exercise 68.—Same as Exercise 67 with the left club—*one—two—three—four.*

Exercise 69.—Double Exercise 67 with the right club. Begin, two front circles reversed—*one—two* ; two side wrist circles reversed—*three—four* ; two back circles reversed—*five—six* ; and two front wrist circles reversed—*seven—eight.*

Exercise 70. —Same as Exercise 69 with the left club.

Exercise 71.—A combination of Exercise 55 and Exercise 61 ; that is, side wrist circle reversed with the right club, and front wrist circle reversed with the left. Hold the clubs as in fig. 84. Do a side wrist circle reversed with the right club, and at the same time a front wrist circle reversed with the left. Count one as the clubs go round. Fig. 122. Same remarks as in Exercise 31.

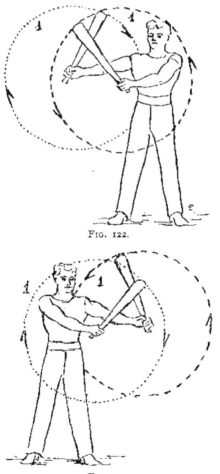

Fig. 122.

Fig. 123.

Exercise 72.—Same kind of exercise as Exercise 71, but this time the left club does a side wrist circle reversed, and the right club at the same time does a front wrist circle reversed. The clubs are held on the left side. Fig. 123.

Exercise 73.—A combination of Exercise 51, Exercise 71, and Exercise 72. It is also a combination of Exercise 67 and Exercise 68.

Same remarks about this exercise as about Exercise 33.

After the first half of Exercise 51, fig. 110, do Exercise 71, fig. 122, and after the second half of Exercise 51, fig. 112, do Exercise 72, fig. 123. Start as in fig. 110 ; front circle reversed with the right, *at the same time* doing a back circle reversed with the left—*one* ; when this is done, the clubs, instead of being in position of fig. 111, must in this case be held a little to the right as in fig. 124, then straighten the arms to the right as

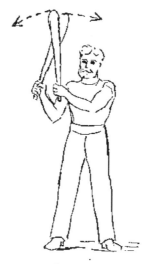

FIG. 124.

in fig. 122, doing *almost at the same time* Exercise 71—*two*—after which resume position of fig. 124; then front circle reversed with the left, and *at the same time* back circle reversed with the right, fig. 112—*three*—

H

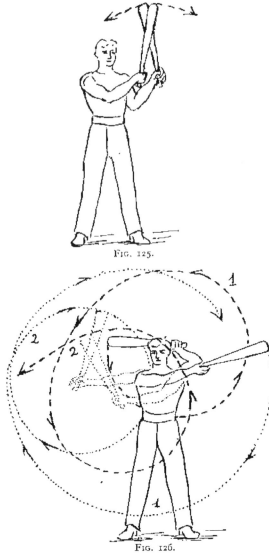

FIG. 125.

FIG. 126.

after which the position is fig. 125, the clubs being held a little to the left.
Now straighten the arms to the left, and do Exercise 72, fig. 123—*tour.*
After this resume position of fig. 125, and begin the exercise again.

Fig. 126 shows times—*one* and *two* of this exercise.

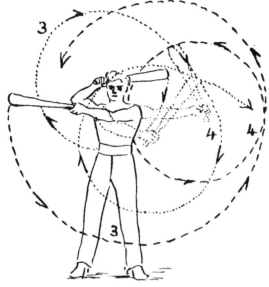

FIG. 127.

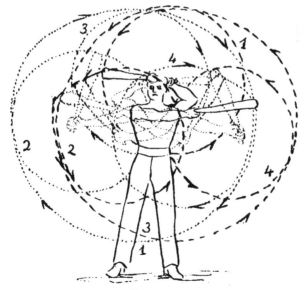

FIG. 128.

Fig. 127 shows times—*three* and *four* of the exercise.

Fig. 128 shows the whole exercise.

Exercise 74.—Double Exercise 73. This ought to be well understood and needs no details.—A reference to Exercise 34 will give a sufficient idea of what is to be done. Time—*one* to *eight*.

Exercise 75.—A combination of Exercise 43 and Exercise 73, fig. 103 and fig. 128. It will be seen that this is simply Exercise 73, to which is added Exercise 43 after each half of the exercise ; that is, after fig. 126 and after fig. 127. In other words, it is the same kind of exercise as Exercise 53, fig. 115. Time—*one* to *six*.

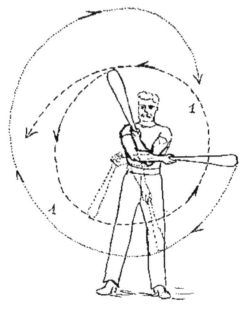

Fig. 129.

Exercise 76.—Front circle reversed and front wrist circle reversed combined, with each club alternately. Begin by a front circle reversed with the right club, and at the same time do a front wrist circle reversed with the left club—*one*, fig. 129.

This figure shows the position just after starting, and the dotted clubs in the figure indicate the position when nearly half of the circles have been done.

When the circles are completed bend the right arm and straighten the left; then do a front wrist circle reversed with the right, and a front circle reversed with the left. Fig. 130—*two.*

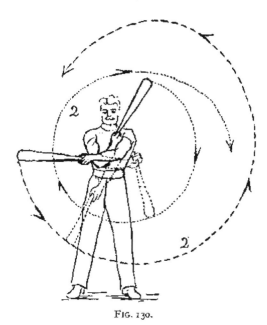

FIG. 130.

The dotted circles of fig. 130 begin where those of fig. 129 finish, so that by looking at both figures the whole course of the clubs during this exercise can be followed easily.

Exercise 77.—A combination of Exercise 76, Exercise 71 and Exercise 72. Start as in the previous exercise, but after time—*one,* fig. 129, do Exercise 71, fig. 122; then do time—*two* of Exercise 76, fig. 130, after which do Exercise 72, fig. 123.   Time—*one—two—three—four.*

Exercise 78.—Double Exercise 77.   Time—*one to eight.*

Exercise 79.—Front circle reversed with one club, doing at *the same time* a side wrist circle reversed, and a back circle reversed with the other. This exercise is the same as Exercise 51, to which is added a side wrist circle reversed, which is done by the club that is executing the back circle reversed, but the side wrist circle reversed is done before the back circle reversed. Begin as in Exercise 51, but the right club must do the front circle reversed in *slower* time, so that whilst it is doing that front circle reversed the left club has time to do, first a side wrist circle reversed, then a back circle reversed. For the same reason the left club must be worked *rather sharply*, so that the back circle reversed is completed at the same time that the other club finishes the front circle reversed. This first part of the exercise is shown by fig. 131. Time— *one, two.*

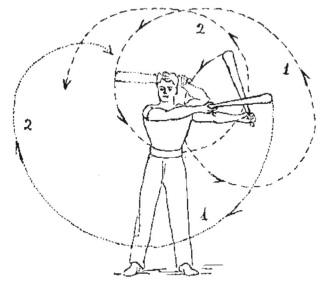

FIG. 131.

When both clubs have completed the circles as above described, the left club does a front circle reversed, whilst the right club does, at *the same time*, a side wrist circle reversed—*three*, and a back circle reversed— *four*. This second part of the exercise is shown in fig. 132.

The whole exercise is shown in fig. 133.

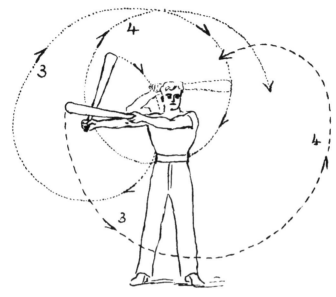

FIG. 132.

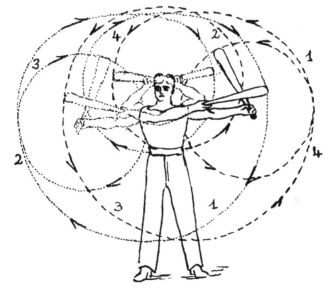

FIG. 133.

Exercise 80.—Front circle reversed, with one club doing at the same time with the other firstly a back circle reversed, and secondly a front wrist circle reversed.   The directions as to the time are exactly the same as in the preceding exercise.   Begin front circle reversed with the right club, doing *at the same time* with the left, first a back circle reversed, counting—*one,* and then a front circle reversed—*two.*   Fig. 134 shows this part of the exercise.

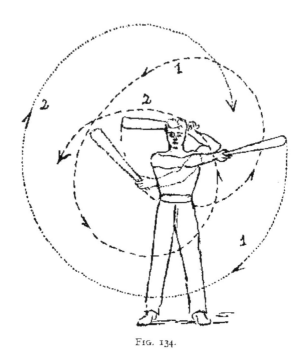

FIG. 134.

Now do a front circle reversed with the left, and, *at the same time* with the right, first a back circle reversed—*three,* after which, a front wrist circle reversed—*four.*   This part of the exercise is shown in fig. 135.

Do not forget that one club, having to do two circles whilst the other only does one, must go quicker, and the other slower.

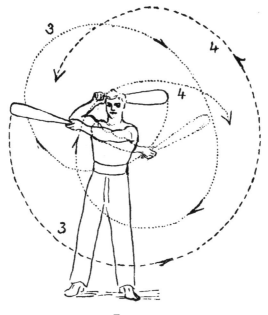

FIG. 135.

I have so far brought the second series to the same level as the first. As in the first series, it has been done gradually. Again I must impress the fact that the club never once changes the direction it is going in, whatever the circle may be. This is clearly shown by fig. 136. The remainder of the Second Series will be found further on.

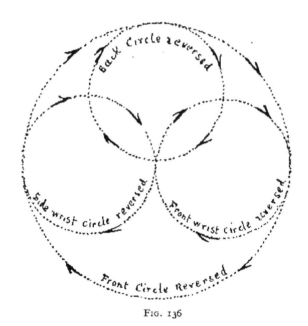

FIG. 136

THIRD SERIES.

The third series, as already explained, is a combination of the first and second. If the clubs are thrown from the right to the left, the right club does the first series and the left the second. If, on the contrary, the clubs are thrown from the left to the right, then the right club does the second series, and the left club the first.

In this third series I shall keep the same order and succession of exercises that I have done in the first and second series, as it will greatly help the learner. I shall also endeavour to avoid too lengthy explanations, as they are apt to confuse. What must be clearly understood is that when in the third series one club does a circle of the first series the other club *always* does a circle of the second series, and *vice versâ.*

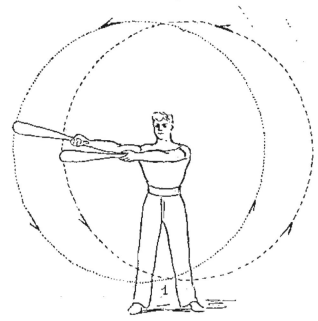

FIG. 137.

Having given all the necessary details in the exercises of the first and second series, it would be superfluous to repeat them in this.

Of course, in the third series, *both* clubs are *always* used. The principal difficulty in this series is to avoid knocking the clubs together. It is easily prevented by letting the club doing the reversed circles go *very slightly* in advance of the other, but this must be done so slightly as not to be noticeable.

Here I must again refer the pupil to the table at the end of the book with regard to the order in which I recommend the exercises to be learned.

Exercise 81.—Front circles. Start to the right, as in fig. 137. Front circle with the right club, and front circle reversed with the left —count *one* as the clubs go round.

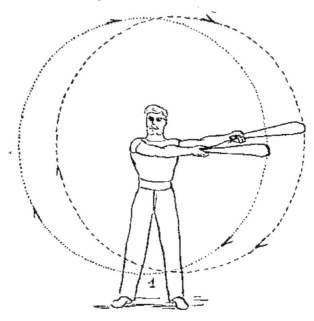

F1G. 138.

Exercise 82.—Same as 81, but start to the left, as in fig. 138. Front circle with the left club, front circle reversed with the right —count *one*.

(From these two first exercises the whole principle of the third series can be easily understood.)

Exercise 83.—Front circlesand back circles com bined. Start to the right, front circles as in Exercise 81—count *one* ; after these

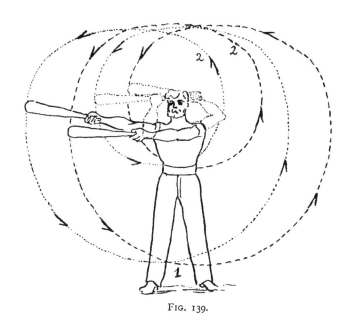

FIG. 139.

bend the arms point the end of both clubs well to the right, and do with the right club a back circle and with the left, *at the same time*, a back circle reversed—count *two*. Fig. 139.

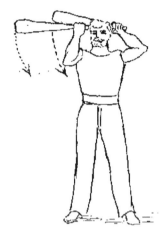

FIG. 140.

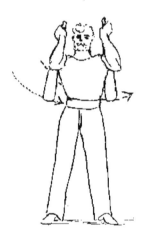

FIG. 141.

The exact motion of the clubs, with position of the arms in doing
the back circles, is shown; the beginning in fig. 140, the middle in
fig. 141, and the end in fig. 142.

Fig. 139 shows the whole exercise.

Exercise 84.—Double Exercise 83, by doing two consecutive
sets of front circles—*one—two*, and two consecutive sets of back
circles—*three—four*.

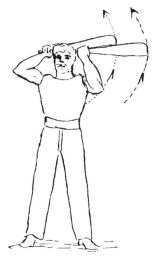

FIG. 142.

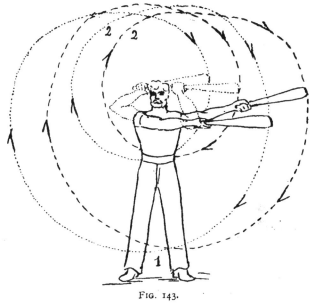

FIG. 143.

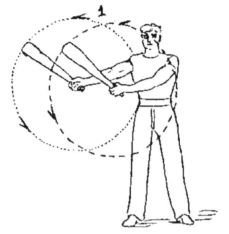

FIG. 144.

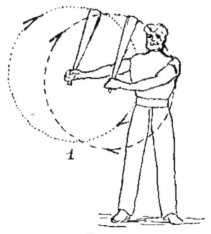

FIG. 145.

Exercise 85.—The same as Exercise 83, but starting to the left.

nt circles as in Exercise 82—count *one*; after which bend the arms, point the end of both clubs well to the left, and do with the right arm a back circle reversed, and with the left, *at the same time*, a back circle—count *two*. Fig. 143.

Exercise 86.—Double Exercise 85.

Exercise 87.—Wrist circles. Hold the clubs out to the right, as in fig. 144.

In this position do a side wrist circle with the right club, and a front wrist circle reversed with the left, count—*one* as the clubs go round.

Exercise 88.—Reverse Exercise 87. Hold the clubs in the same manner, but do a side wrist circle reversed with the right club, and a front wrist circle with the left, both, of course, *at the same time.* Fig. 145.

It will be seen that the clubs go exactly in the opposite direction to that of Exercise 87.

Exercise 89.—Same as Exercise 87, but holding the clubs to the left instead of the right. In that position it is the right club that does a front wrist circle reversed, the left doing this time a side wrist circle—count *one.*

Time—*three* of fig. 147 shows this exercise.

Exercise 90.—Reverse Exercise 89. Hold the clubs in the same manner to the left; side wrist circle reversed with the left and front wrist circle with the right—*one.*

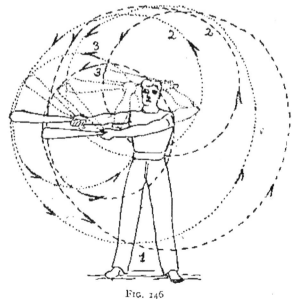

Fig. 146

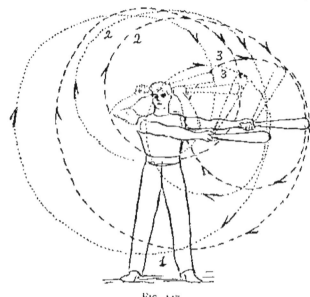

FIG. 147.

Time—*two* of fig. 148 shows this exercise.

Exercise 91.—A combination of Exercises 83 and 87. Do the Exercise 83 entirely, fig. 139, but after the back circles hold out the clubs as in Exercise 87, fig. 144, and do the wrist circles described in Exercise 87. The arms need not be held out perfectly straight; this would look rather stiff. Bend them slightly; it looks better, and renders the exercise easier. Of course, after having done the wrist circles the clubs are thrown downwards to begin again the front circles. The time is, front circles—*one*; back circles—*two*; wrist circles—*three*. Fig. 146 shows this exercise.

Exercise 92.—Double Exercise 91. Time—*one* to *six*.

Exercise 93.—Same as Exercise 91, but starting to the left instead of the right. A combination of Exercises 85 and 89. Do Exercise 85 entirely, fig. 143; after which do the wrist circles as in Exercise 89. The whole of this exercise is shown in fig. 147. Time, *one—two—three*.

Exercise 94.—Double Exercise 93.   Time, *one* to *six.*

Exercise 95.—A combination of Exercises 83 and 90.   In this exercise the wrist circles are done between the front circles and the back circles of Exercise 83.   Begin as in Exercise 83 by doing front circles, but when the clubs are at the left, as shown in fig. 148, do the wrist

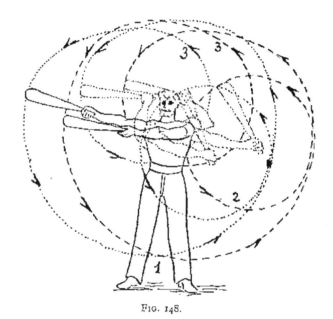

FIG. 148.

circles described in Exercise 90, after which continue the upward direction of the clubs and do back circles as in Exercise 83.   Time, front circles—*one*; wrist circles—*two*; back circles—*three.*   This exercise is shown in fig. 148.

Exercise 96.—Double Exercise 95.   Time, *one* to *six.*

Exercise 97.—The same as Exercise 95, but starting to the left instead of the right.   A combination of Exercises 85 and 88.   Start as in Exercise 85, doing front circles; when the clubs arrive at the

I 2

right side, do the wrist circles of Exercise 88; after which do the back circles of Exercise 85. Time, *one—two—three.*   Fig. 149 shows this exercise.

Exercise 98.—Double Exercise 97.   Time, *one to six.*

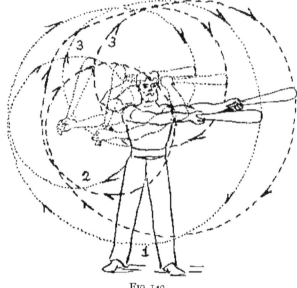

FIG 149.

Exercise 99.—A combination of Exercises 87 and 95.   Do entirely Exercise 95, fig. 148, but after the back circles are done, when the clubs are going to begin again the front circles, extend the arms to the right and do the wrist circles of Exercise 87, fig. 144. The time is, starting to the right, front circles—*one ;* wrist circles at the left side—*two ;* back circles—*three ;* and wrist circles at the right side—*four.*   The whole exercise is shown in fig. 150.

It may be noticed that this exercise is also a combination of Exercises 90 and 91.

To show the correctness of the method I have employed throughout this book, I shall just point out that the Exercise 99 is an exact combination of Exercises 27 and 68.   The right club does Exercise 27, which belongs to the First Series, and the left club does Exercise 68, which belongs to the Second Series.

Exercise 100.—Double Exercise 99—*one* to *eight.*

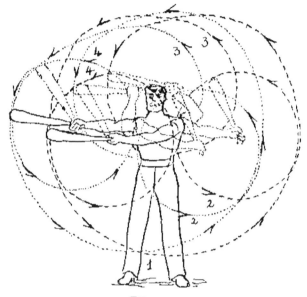

FIG. 150.

Exercise 101.—Same as Exercise 99, but starting to the left instead of to the right. It is Exercise 97, to which is added Exercise 89. Do entirely Exercise 97, fig. 149, but after the back circles hold the clubs to the left and do the wrist circles of Exercise 89. Time—*one* to *four.* The whole exercise is shown in fig. 151.

Exercise 102.—Double Exercise 101—*one* to *eight.*

So far I have embodied in the Third Series most of the exercises already described of the First and Second Series. These exercises, from Exercise 81 to Exercise 102, have been done by using the clubs in such a manner that they both go together at the same time, describing circles of the same category, although one circle is ordinary and the other reversed. Now, all the circles and combinations of these exercises, from Exercise 83 to Exercise 102, can also be done by separating the clubs, so that one

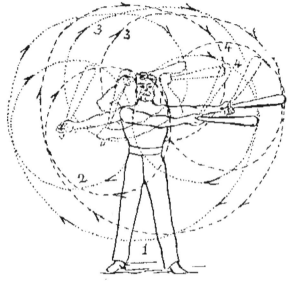

FIG 151.

works in advance of the other.   After Exercise 86, I mentioned that the
club doing the reversed circles should go slightly in advance of the
other.   To effect what I mean by separating the clubs, all that is
required is, that the club doing the reversed circles should go—*one
time*—*in advance of the other.*   That very simple alteration will at once
enable the pupil to do exercises which to the uninitiated appear most
intricate.   This fact once well remembered, it will be most easy to
understand the few following exercises.   In fact, they are a mere
repetition of Exercises 83 to 102, but done in the way just mentioned.
I shall, however, give these new exercises numbers, this being useful for
reference; besides, they are really quite distinct exercises by themselves.
I leave out Exercise 81 and Exercise 82, as they cannot well be done in
this way.

Exercise 103.—Front circles and back circles combined, starting to
the right, that is to say, the same as Exercise 83, but done in the manner
described above.

The clubs must both be kept going, *without stopping*, all through the exercise. First try the exercise slowly, following my directions and the figures, but when once the exercise is understood there must be no stopping whatever, all going smoothly and in time.

Clubs in the starting position, throw the left club first, beginning a front circle reversed, as in fig. 152.

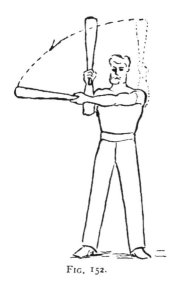

Fig. 152.

When the left club passes the legs count—*one*, and then throw the right club downwards, beginning a front circle, the clubs then getting into the position shown in fig. 153.

When the right club passes the legs count—*two*. Both clubs continue their course upwards, right following left, and before time—*three*, they are in the position shown in fig. 154.

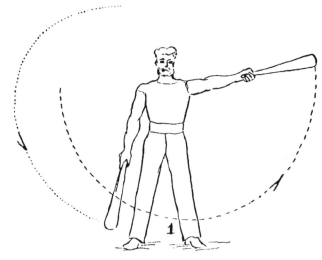

FIG. 153.

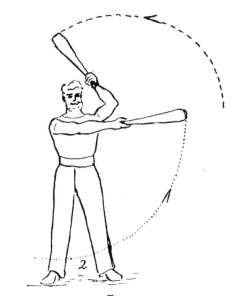

FIG. 154.

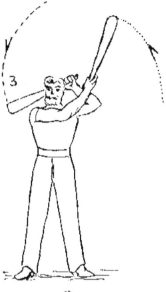

FIG. 155.

Then do a back circle reversed with the left, counting—*three*, and getting at the same time the right club ready for a back circle. This position is shown in fig. 155.

When the left club has completed the back circle reversed, do the back circle with the right, counting —*four*, and bringing at the same time the left club in position to start again, as in the dotted clubs of fig. 152. The last position of the clubs is shown by fig. 156.

After the above position, fall again into that of fig. 152, and so on. The whole course taken by the clubs is shown by fig. 139, Exercise 83, which is exactly what the clubs are doing in Exercise 103, but they are separated, that is to say, follow one another instead of working together.

I have detailed this Exercise 103 somewhat at length, in order that the pupil may understand well how this class of exercise is done, though I believe my previous remarks are quite sufficient to convey clearly what I mean. It must also be noticed that a circle with one club does not begin until the circle that is being done by the other is almost finished. The

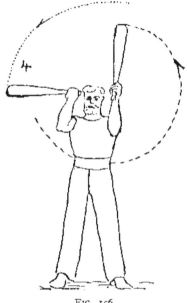

FIG. 156.

circles are *not done together,* but follow one another, as already stated.
That is the reason why Exercise 103 is composed of four " times," whilst
Exercise 83, of which Exercise 103 is a repetition, with clubs separated, is
only composed of two. All this must be well understood, as it would
take so much space if I had to detail every exercise of this class, as I
have done Exercise 103. The great secret is that the club doing the
reversed circles goes first, one time ahead of the other.

Exercise 104.—Same as Exercise 103, starting to the left. The
right club leads. This time the right club does the reversed circles, and
the left the ordinary circles. Bear this in mind for all exercises of this
class done when starting to the left.

Exercise 105.—Front circles, back circles, and wrist circles done
on the right side, with clubs separated, starting to the right. This exercise is the same as Exercise 91, but separating the clubs. The left club
leads. Time—*one* to *six.*

Exercise 106.—Same as Exercise 105, starting to the left. The right club leads.—*One to six.*

Exercise 107.—Front circles, wrist circles done on the left side, and back circles, starting to the right. Same as in Exercise 95, but separating the clubs. The left club leads. Time—*one to six.*

Exercise 108.—Same as Exercise 107, starting to the left. The right club leads.—*One to six.*

Exercise 109.—A combination of Exercises 105 and 107, starting to the right. Front circles and wrist circles done on the left, back circles and wrist circles done on the right. It is Exercise 99 done with clubs separated. The left club leads. Time—*one to eight.*

Exercise 110.—The same as Exercise 109, starting to the left. The right club leads.—*One to eight.*

This last exercise finishes what I may call the simple regular exercises of the Third Series. There are, however, a good many more which come under this series, but in most of these the circles done by the right club are generally of an entirely different class to those done by the left, though keeping the rule hitherto observed as regards series; that is to say, if one club does a simple circle, the other club will do a reversed circle, although this reversed circle may not be of the corresponding class to the simple circle. For instance, until now in the Third Series, when the right club has been doing a back circle, the left did a back circle reversed, or, as in the last exercises, the left followed immediately with a back circle reversed; but in some of the following exercises, when the right club is doing a back circle, the left may be doing a front circle reversed, or a wrist circle reversed. I shall now describe a few of these exercises, which, after the foregoing explanations, ought to be easily understood.

Exercise 111.—Front circle reversed with the left club, and back circle with the right.

Start to the right, both clubs doing the circles at the same time. Both circles must be begun and finished together. Count—*one*—as the clubs go round. Do not forget that they are no longer separated. Fig. 157 shows this exercise.

Exercise 112.—Same as Exercise 111, but start to the left, the left club doing the back circle, and the right club the front circle reversed—*one.*

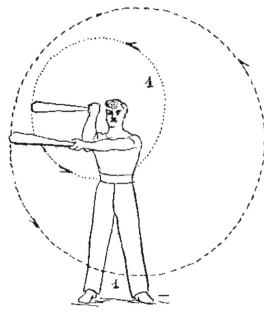

FIG. 157.

Exercise 113.—Front circle with the right club and back circle reversed with the left.

Start to the right, both clubs doing the circles at the same time; count—*one.* Fig. 158.

Exercise 114.—Same as Exercise 113, but start to the left, left club doing a front circle, and the right club a back circle reversed—*one.*

Exercise 115.—A combination of Exercise 111 and Exercise 113, or perhaps, more correctly, alternately, first one then the other. Start as in Exercise 111 ; do that exercise entirely through once, but when ready to begin again, do Exercise 113. When Exercise 113 has been done entirely once, begin another Exercise 111, and so on. Thus the right arm does a back circle and a front circle—that is, Exercise 5 of the First Series— whilst the left arm is doing a front circle reversed and a back circle reversed—that is, Exercise 46 of the Second Series ; only notice that when one club is doing a back circle the other is doing a front circle. This exercise must be done neatly and without hurry. Fig. 159 shows the exercise. Time—*one—two.*

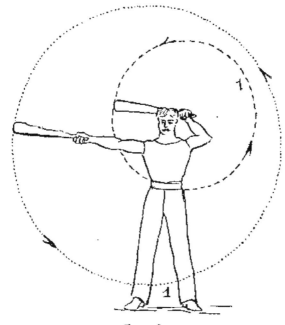

FIG. 158.

Exercise 116.—Same as Exercise 115, but starting to the left, being Exercise 112 and Exercise 114 combined—*one—two.*

Exercise 117.—Front circle reversed and back circle reversed with the left club, doing *at the same time*, with each circle, a back circle with the right club.

Start as in Exercise 111, doing that exercise entirely, count—*one*—but immediately after do a back circle reversed with the left, still doing another back circle with the right, count—*two.* It will perhaps be clearer if I say that the left club does Exercise 46, whilst the right club keeps on doing the back circle with each circle done by the left. Fig. 160 shows this exercise.

Exercise 118.—Same as Exercise 117, but starting to the left. In this exercise it is the left club that does the back circles whilst the right does the front circle reversed and the back circle reversed. Count—*one—two.*

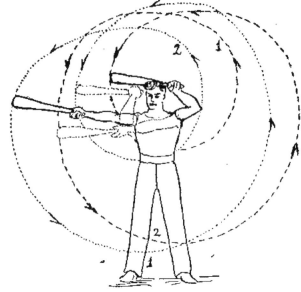

FIG. 159.

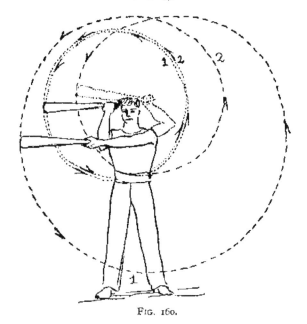

FIG. 160.

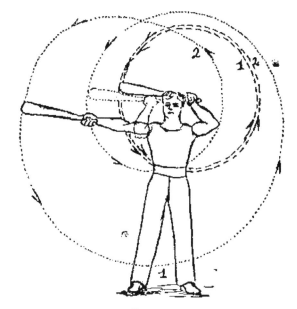

FIG. 161.

Exercise 119.—Front circle and back circle with the right club, the left doing a back circle reversed at each circle done by the right.

Start as in Exercise 113 do that exercise entirely, but before beginning it again do a back circle with the right, doing at the same time a back circle reversed with the left. Time—*one—two.* This exercise is Exercise 5 done with the right club, the left doing at the same time back circles reversed. Fig. 161 shows this exercise.

Exercise 120.—Same as Exercise 119, but starting to the left. The left club does a front circle and a back circle, the right doing at the same time back circles reversed—*one—two.*

In this first part I have introduced all the principal and regular exercises of the First, Second and Third Series, but of course from them many others may be done with some slight alterations or by combining them together.

I may here again repeat that the 120 foregoing exercises are merely combinations of eight of the Key Exercises or Circles and this might even be simplified by saying that they are combinations of the four first circles, these circles being in some exercises reversed. Thus it will be seen that the most difficult exercises of the 120 already described, being only combinations of such simple circles as the Key Circles, ought really to be easily learned and done, if all the exercises have been gone through in rotation as given.

Now I am going to introduce the two last circles of the Key, viz., the lower back circle and the lower back circle reversed. Though these names may not sound quite elegant to some ears, I have given them to those circles because they best convey their meaning.

These circles, together with the combinations and exercises formed with them, and also some other miscellaneous exercises not included in the preceding 120, will form the second part of this book.

Second Part.

CHAPTER III.

I HAVE already explained at the end of the last chapter what this second part will include, and I shall now proceed to describe the Nos. 5 and 10 of the Key exercises. These two circles, to which I have given the names of lower back circle and lower back circle reversed, have only been known for the last few years, that is to say, about thirteen years, and I think I may say that, as far as I know, I have introduced them in London. They possibly may have been known before that time, for there really is "nothing new under the sun." However, I do not believe they were seen in London until introduced by me at the German Gymnasium some twelve or thirteen years ago, and I remember their creating quite a sensation at St. James's Hall, where, assisting at one of the London Athletic Club's Assaults-of-Arms, I did some lower back circles with a 44lbs. club. Previous to that I had never seen the exercise done by anyone, whether amateur or professional, and I know that if used at present it is only subsequent to my having introduced it as already mentioned, and my having taught it even to very good club performers, several of them professionals, who, though they had often seen me doing it, could not quite make out how it was done. Therein lies the difficulty, though I may say at once that, when the knack of it is acquired, it is really easier than a common back circle. It has also the advantage of being easy of combination with the 120 exercises described in the first part of this book, but to do this, the pupil must be perfect in those 120 exercises, so as to be able to devote the whole of his attention to combining the lower back circles with them, and this is why I have until now delayed introducing these circles; besides, only an already proficient person can thoroughly understand those combinations. ĸ

Lower Back Circle (figs. 5 and 162) with the right club. Throw the club as when doing a front circle. See dotted arm and club in fig. 162. Here I must remark that doing a lower back circle only,

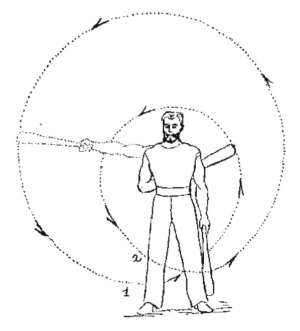

Fig. 162.

as in fig. 5, several times in succession, would be too difficult for any beginner, and for that reason I have made use of the front circle, thus rendering the lower back circle much easier. That explains the difference between fig. 5 and fig. 162. Particular attention must now be paid to the elbow, as in that lies all the secret of the circle, the same as in the case with the ordinary back circles. When the club gets down by the side of the right leg, bend the arm slightly, the elbow going a little in advance of the hand and club, as shown in fig. 163. From that position the elbow does not move, that is, does not go higher, but it turns a little, and the hand and club continue

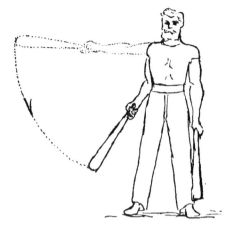

FIG. 163.

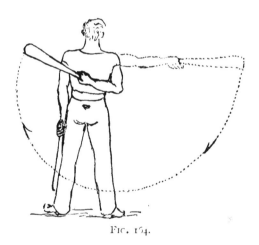

FIG. 164.

their course behind the back, the forearm alone being moved in doing so, until the position attained is as in fig. 162. The back view of that position is shown in fig. 164.

Here particularly notice the position of the hand. It is in the middle of the back, between the shoulder-blades, the knuckles are outwards, the nails turned inwards against the back.

K 2

To complete the circle, the wrist is turned so that the knuckles go inwards against the back and the nails come outwards. The position is then as shown in fig. 165.

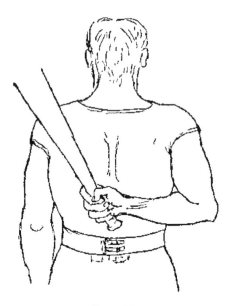

·FIG. 165.

At the same time the elbow comes forward, the hand and club following it. Fig. 166.

Continue the circle by bringing the elbow forward to position of fig. 167.

Here notice the position of the elbow, which has come quite forward. The shoulder is also necessarily forward. To finish the circle the hand passes by the hip-bone, as in fig. 167, and drops down to the position

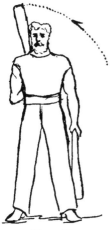

FIG. 166.

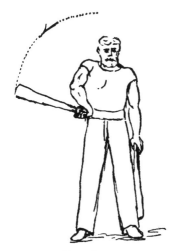

FIG. 167.

shown by the dotted arm in fig. 168.   The elbow must be kept forward.
Then the arm is straightened and the front circle continued as shown
by the dotted circle in fig. 168 until arrived at the position of the dotted
arm and club in fig. 162, where the circle begins.

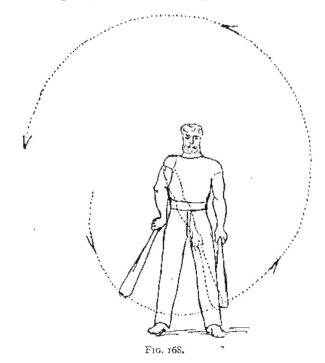

Fig. 168.

In the last three figures, Nos. 166, 167, 168, the shoulder should be
leant forward, and a slight turn of the body towards the left will greatly
assist, but this must not be exaggerated.

This detailed description of the lower back circle must necessarily
appear rather complicated, it but must be read holding at the same time
a club in the hand, following with it the directions given, and getting in
the right position by the aid of the figures.   If this is done slowly several
times, I have no doubt that this circle will be soon learnt.   Working
before a looking-glass will greatly assist.   The whole course of the club
is shown in fig. 162.

Do the same exercise with the left arm. Of course the directions are the same as for the right arm.

Lower Back Circle Reversed with the right club. Fig. 10 and fig. 169.

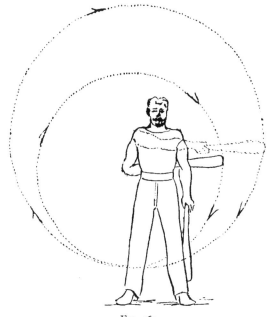

FIG. 169.

This exercise should not be tried until the lower back circle is fully mastered.

The lower back circle reversed is so correctly and completely the preceding exercise *reversed*, that for its description I shall make use of the figures given for the lower back circle, beginning with the last and finishing with the first. Really the best way to learn the lower back circle reversed is to do a lower back circle rather slowly, and, instead of straightening the arm when finishing, as in fig. 168, to keep it bent and *slowly take the club back the way it came.* If this be done correctly the lower back circle reversed will have been done.

In the lower back circle reversed the elbow *follows* the club and the hand.

Start as shown by dotted arm in fig. 169, that is to say, a front circle
reversed.   Bend the arm as in fig. 168, elbow being kept well forward,
shoulder also leaning forward.   From this position the club goes up to
position of fig. 167; from there to that of fig. 166, then to that of fig.
165.   Now pay attention to the turn of the hand; turn the wrist so
that the knuckles come outwards and the nails inwards against the
back, thus getting into the position of fig. 164, which is also that of fig.
169.   From there the club goes down passing behind the left and the
right leg, until it gets into the position of fig. 163, after which straighten
the arm and continue the front circle reversed upwards to the position
of the dotted arm in fig. 169.   This figure shows the whole exercise.
Of course when looking at the figures 163 to 168 it must not be forgotten
that in the lower back circle reversed the direction the club is going in is
exactly the reverse to that marked in those figures; this can easily be
seen by following the dotted circles of fig. 169.

Do the lower back circle reversed with the left arm.   Same directions.

Now that the pupil is supposed to have learnt the two remaining
circles of the Key, I shall introduce them in the following chapter, giving
them numbers for reference.

CHAPTER IV.

I HAVE already said that the lower back circle and the lower back circle reversed can be introduced and combined with most of the 120 exercises described in the first part. I shall now show how this can be done, but after the first few exercises of each series, I shall merely name the exercises, giving them numbers for reference, as any lengthened details would be a mere repetition of what has already been written. After the first few exercises, the principle of the combinations must be perfectly understood, as, if I were to describe every exercise minutely, it would unnecessarily enlarge this book without giving a corresponding benefit to the pupil. I am doing my best for him, but I must beg him to do his best for me by thoroughly learning first the Key exercises in the rotation given, then the exercises in the order recommended by me in the table at the end of the book. If he has done so he will now be able to do most of the following exercises without my having to give him all the details over again.

First Series—Second Part.

Exercise 121.—Front circle and lower back circle with the right club, fig. 162. This has been fully described. Count—*one* after having done the first half of the front circle, and—*two* after the lower back circle. See fig. 162.

Exercise 122.—Same as Exercise 121, but with the left club—*one* —*two*.

Exercise 123.—Do alternately Exercise 121 and Exercise 122, with both clubs, using them both at the same time. This exercise will be better understood if I remark that it is the same style of exercise as Exercise 11, doing, of course, a lower back circle instead of a back circle.

Start as if going to do Exercise 3, fig. 59. The right club goes behind
the back to do a lower back circle, and the left club begins at the same
time a front circle, both assuming the position shown in fig. 170; continuing

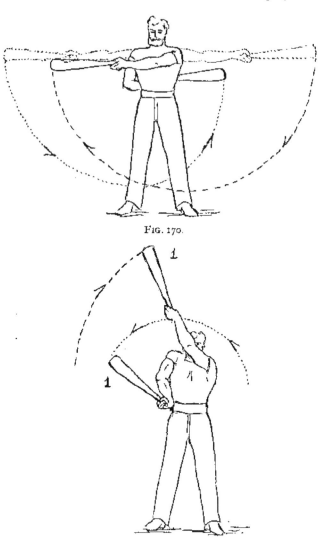

Fig. 170.

Fig. 171.

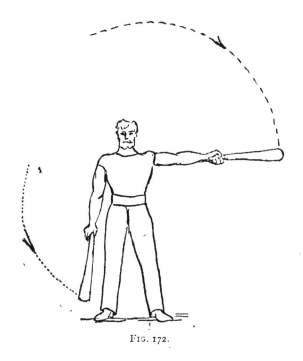

FIG. 172.

the circles, the clubs are as in fig. 171. At this position count—*one,* then, completing the circles, the position is as in fig. 172.

Now the left club goes down to do a lower back circle, the right club continuing its course to complete a front circle, as shown in fig. 173.

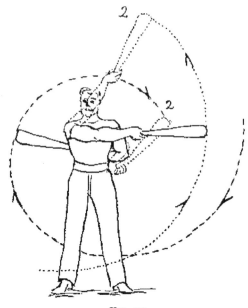

FIG. 173.

When arrived in the position of the dotted clubs in fig. 173, count—*two.* Then the right club goes down to the right to do the lower back circle, and the left club goes down to the left to do a front circle, thus beginning again, then getting in the fully-drawn position of fig. 170, and so on. The extending of both arms, as shown by the dotted arms in the said figures, is done only when *first* starting the exercise; but afterwards the starting position is more like that of fig. 172—that is to say, as to starting to the left; when starting to the right the left arm is down and the right arm extended.

The whole exercise is shown in fig. 174.

Of course, the entire exercise must be done without any stoppage; if I have divided it, it is to make it easier to learn.

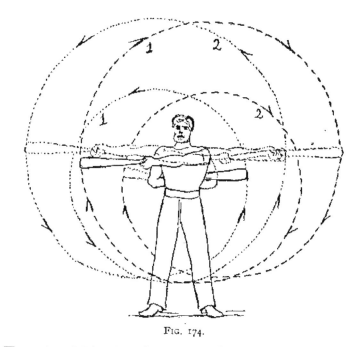

FIG. 174.

Exercise 124.—Exercise 121 combined with a back circle with the right club.

Start exactly as in Exercise 121, but when arrived at the position, or rather a little farther than the position of the dotted arm in fig. 168, instead of beginning another front circle, bend the arm upwards and do a back circle exactly as in Exercise 5, fig. 63. Exercise 124 is shown in fig. 175. Time—front circle—*one;* lower back circle—*two;* back circle—*three.*

Exercise 125.—Same as Exercise 124 with the left club.

Exercise 126.—A combination of Exercise 11 and Exercise 123. Also similar to Exercise 124 and Exercise 125, done alternately. Start a front circle with the right club, doing at the same time a back circle with the left; when the right club gets close to the right leg, instead of continuing the front circle, do a lower back circle with the right, and with the left do another back circle. It will be seen

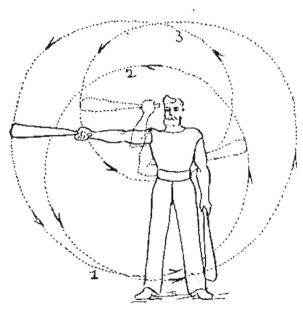

FIG. 175.

that the left club does two consecutive back circles, whilst the right does part of a front circle and a lower back circle, which is exactly the same as Exercise 121. The circles done by both arms are shown in fig. 176, this forming the first part of the exercise.

The lower back circle with the right club is done between the two back circles of the left club. The first back circle must be finished just when the right club passes behind the right leg, and the second back circle finishes just after the right club is extended, as in dotted arm of fig. 168. The whole movement is like a quick time of three, *one* for the first left back circle, *two* for the right lower back circle, and *three* for the second left back circle. Of course this is not the right counting for the exercise, but I give it just to convey a better idea of the respective time of the circles. The reason why two back circles are done instead of only one is to avoid the clubs clashing together, or the knocking of the left elbow with the right club.

The proper time for counting is—*one*—after the first back circle, and—*two*—after the second. This completes the first part of the exercise, that is, fig. 176. When finishing the circles, as far as they are indicated in that figure, the clubs are in the position shown in fig. 177.

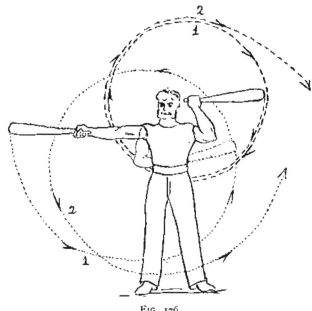

FIG. 176.

Now the right club goes sharply upwards and does a back circle; the left club goes down doing a lower back circle, and the right club does another back circle, counting—*three* and *four*. Of course the directions as to the time of doing the circles are the same as for the first part of the exercise.

The second part is shown by fig. 178.

Exercise 127.—Same as Exercise 126, but adding the wrist circles exactly as done in Exercise 33, figs. 89, 90, 91. Time—*one* to *six*.

Exercise 128.—Same kind of exercise as Exercise 126, only instead of doing the two back circles do first a front wrist circle and then a back circle as in Exercises 23 and 24, figs. 80 and 81. The lower back circle comes, as before, *between* the front wrist circle and the back circle. In other respects the way of doing the exercise is the same as Exercise 126. Same time.

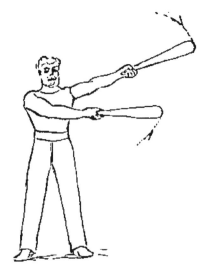

FIG. 177.

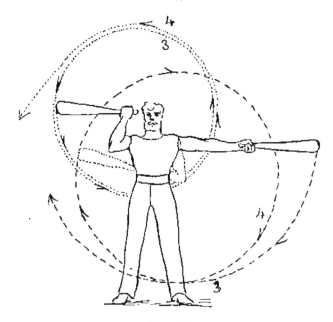

FIG. 178.

Exercise 129.—Same as Exercise 128, but with the addition of the wrist circles, as in Exercise 127. *One to six.*

Exercise 130.—A combination of Exercise 9 and lower back circles. It is exactly Exercise 9, fig. 66, to which is added after time—*one*—the lower back circle done with both clubs *at the same time,* counting—*two,* after which do back circles with both arms as in Exercise 9. Count—*three.* This Exercise 130 is shown in fig. 179. It will be noticed that it is also

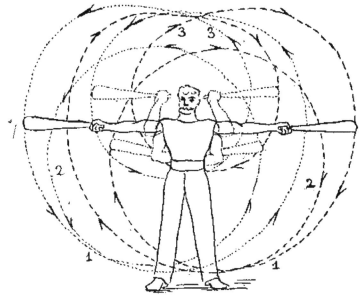

FIG. 179.

Exercises 124 and 125 done simultaneously with both arms. It is difficult to do this exercise well. Though I might give a few more exercises of this class I think that for all purposes those I have introduced will prove sufficient; the pupil may add to them any others that his ingenuity may suggest; he may, for instance, double those I have given. I shall now proceed to the exercises of the same description belonging to the second series. They will be given exactly in the same order as those of the first series, being merely their reversed motion.

L

SECOND SERIES—SECOND PART.

Exercise 131.—Front circle reversed and lower back circle reversed with the right club. Fig. 169. This has already been described. Count—*one*—after the first half of the front circle reversed, and —*two*—after the lower back circle reversed.

Exercise 132.—Same as Exercise 131, with the left club—*one*—*two*.

Exercise 133.—Alternate Exercises 131 and 132, using both clubs at the same time. This exercise is best done if the right club goes first, and the left club is started only when the right has arrived behind the back in the position shown in fig. 180.

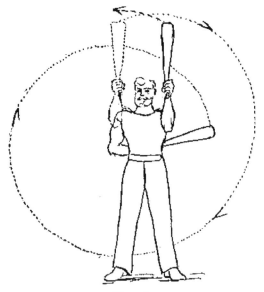

FIG. 180.

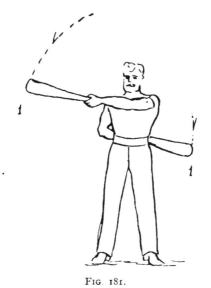

FIG. 181.

In fig. 181 I show the position of both clubs when the left has started, and at this position count—*one*.   After this the clubs continue the circles.

L 2

The left arm does a lower back circle reversed, and the right a front circle reversed, assuming the position shown in fig. 182; that is, the right extended and the left bent behind the back. At this position count—*two.* Fig. 182 shows the whole exercise.

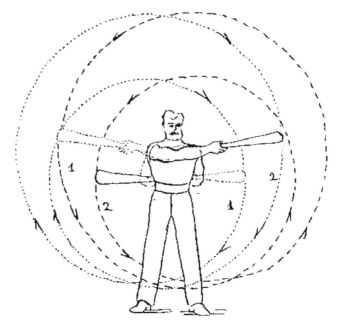

FIG. 182.

Exercise 134.—Exercise 131 combined with a back circle reversed with the right club. Start exactly as in Exercise 131, but after the lower back circle reversed, do a back circle reversed as in Exercise 45, fig. 106. Exercise 134 is shown in Figure 183.

Exercise 135.—Same as Exercise 134, with the left club.

Exercise 136.—A combination of Exercises 51 and 133. Front circle reversed with the right, doing at the same time a back circle reversed with the left—*one;* lower back circle reversed with the right, and back circle reversed with the left—*two.* This forms the first part of the exercise, and is shown in fig. 184. Then front circle reversed with the

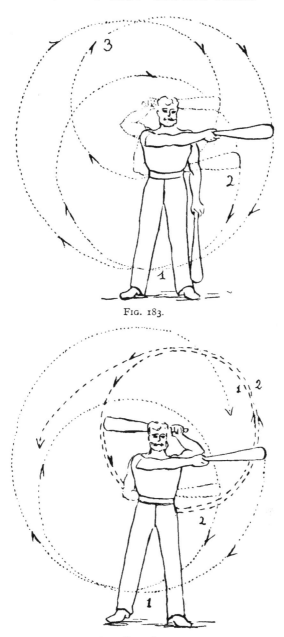

Fig. 183.

Fig. 184.

left, and back circle reversed with the right—*three ;* lower back circle reversed with the left, and back circle reversed with the right—*four.* This is the second part of the exercise, and is shown in fig. 185. Follow exactly the same instructions as in Exercise 126.

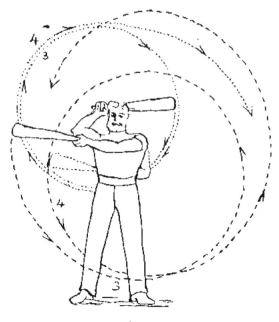

FIG. 185.

Exercise 137.—Same as Exercise 136, but adding the wrist circles exactly as done in Exercise 73, figs. 126, 127 and 128. Time—*one* to *six.*

Exercise 138.—Same kind of exercise as Exercise 136, but instead of doing the two back circles reversed, do first a back circle reversed and then a front wrist circle reversed, as in Exercise 63 and Exercise 64, fig. 120. The lower back circle reversed of one club comes *between* the back circle reversed and the front wrist circle reversed of the other.—*One* to *four.*

Exercise 139.—Same as Exercise 138, with the addition of the wrist circles as in Exercise 137. Time—*one* to *six.*

Exercise 140.—A combination of Exercise 49 and the lower back circle reversed. It is exactly Exercise 49, fig. 109, to which is added after time—*one*—a lower back circle reversed, done with both clubs *at the same time*—counting *two*—after which both clubs do a back circle reversed—*three*. This is also Exercises 134 and 135 done simultaneously with both clubs.

Here finishes the second part of the second series, but, as already remarked, many other exercises can be done besides those here introduced. These can also be doubled.

THIRD SERIES—SECOND PART.

Exercise 141.—Front circle and lower back circle with the right club, doing at the same time a front circle reversed and a lower back circle reversed with the left. A combination of Exercises 121 and 132.

Start with both clubs to the right, as in Exercise 81, fig. 137. When the clubs arrive close to the legs pass them both behind, doing with the right club a lower back circle, and with the left a lower back circle reversed. Count—*one* and *two*. This exercise is not so difficult as it may appear, both clubs going in the same direction. It is the same kind of exercise as Exercise 83, lower back circles being done instead of back circles. A glance at fig. 186, which shows this exercise, will give a much better idea of the exercise than any written description.

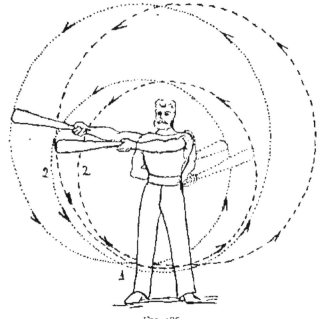

FIG. 186.

Exercise 142.—Same as Exercise 141. Starting to the left instead of to the right. Front circle and lower back circle with the left, and front circle reversed and lower back circle reversed with the right—*one—two.*

Exercise 143.—Same as Exercise 141, but adding to it the back circles after the lower back circles ; that is, combining Exercise 141 with Exercise 83, fig. 139.

Do the whole of Exercise 141, and after the lower back circles, instead of quite finishing the front circles, bend the arms as in Exercise 83 and do the back circles of that exercise, counting—*three,* after which the clubs are again thrown out to begin the Exercise 141.

Fig. 187 shows Exercise 143.

Exercise 144.—Same as Exercise 143, but done starting to the left instead of to the right. This is Exercises 85 and 142 combined.

Exercise 145.—The same as Exercise 143, but adding to it the wrist circles after the back circles, as in Exercise 91, fig. 146.

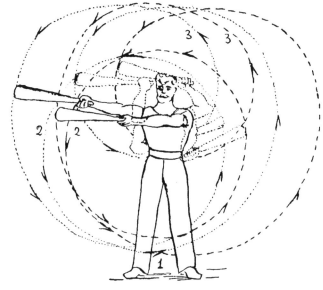

FIG. 187.

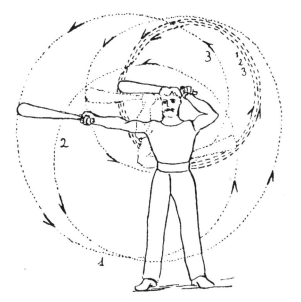

FIG. 188.

Exercise 146.—The same as Exercise 144, adding to it the wrist circles after the back circles, as in Exercise 93, fig. 147.

Exercise 147.—Three back circles reversed in succession with the left club, whilst the right club is doing Exercise 124, fig. 175. When the right club starts to do a front circle, begin a back circle reversed with the left, as in Exercise 113, fig. 158, counting—*one*—whilst doing that first back circle reversed. After this do a lower back circle with the right, and another back circle reversed with the left—*two;* then a back circle with the right, doing at the same time a third back circle reversed with the left —*three*, this last part being the same as the second part of Exercise 83. The lower back circle with the right is done *slightly in advance* of the second back circle reversed with the left; this is to avoid the clashing of the clubs. The exercise is shown in fig. 188.

Exercise 148.—Same as Exercise 147, but done to the left instead of to the right, so that it is the right club that does the back circles reversed, whilst the left does Exercise 125.

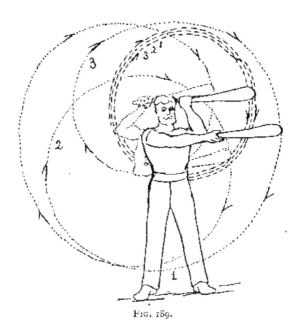

FIG. 189.

Exercise 149.—Three back circles in succession with the left club, whilst the right does Exercise 134, fig. 183. This exercise is exactly of the same kind as Exercise 147, so I need not give further details. It is shown in fig. 189. Time—*one—two—three.*

Eercise 150.—Same as Exercise 149, but done to the left instead of to the right. The right club does the back circles, whilst the left does Exercise 135.

Here, I may say, finish the regular exercises with the Indian clubs, though many more might have been added ; for instance, Exercise 147 can have wrist circles added to it ; it can also be combined in various ways with Exercise 150, all of which are very effective. Again, by a very simple change of the clubs, their being made to change sides by passing them from one shoulder over to the other, you can fall into Exercise 148 and combine with Exercise 149. These can also combine with Exercises 141, 142, 143, and 144, which in turn can produce different combinations by being changed from right to left, and *vice versâ*. Altogether, I may safely say that anyone with a little thought can form nearly 500 combinations out of the 150 exercises which I have introduced and endeavoured to explain to the best of my abilities. It has been a difficult task which could not have been accomplished satisfactorily had I not adopted the system which I have made use of, and which I believe to be the only efficacious one for teaching Indian clubs by means of a book, and, that is, by having a key of five simple circles which form the base of all combinations, however intricate they may be. I have spared no illustrations, especially at the beginning, where the pupil needs more assistance.

I have just said that some new exercises may be done by a simple change of the clubs from one shoulder to the other. Many may wonder what I mean. I will now explain my meaning by here introducing those changes as exercises. They are rather difficult to describe, but I will endeavour to do so as clearly as possible.

These changes are used to pass from one exercise of one series to another exercise of another series without having, in any way, to stop the motion of the clubs ; they are, as it were, a connecting link. With their aid it is possible to go through the whole of the three series without any perceptible stoppage of the clubs, though of course they break and reverse the direction of the swing.

The following are the changes—

Exercise 151.—Change from the first series to the second series with the right club.

Start exactly as when doing Exercise 5, which is done almost entirely, but when half of the back circle has been done, and the club is pointed towards the left shoulder, as shown in fig. 190, stop the upward swing, and instead of finishing the back circle, *sharply* pass your hand (which was close to the right ear—see fig. 190) right over the centre of the head and bring it in the position of the front circle reversed, as shown in fig. 191.

This movement must be done tolerably quickly, so that the club has not time to fall from the position of fig. 190. It merely travels

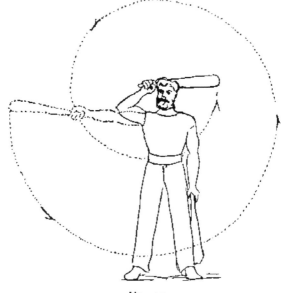

No. 190.

horizontally for a few inches towards the left, and when the arm is straight, as in fig. 191, the club goes down, doing a front circle reversed, thus having changed from the first series to the second series. Fig. 191 gives a good idea of the change.

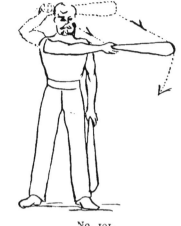

No. 191.

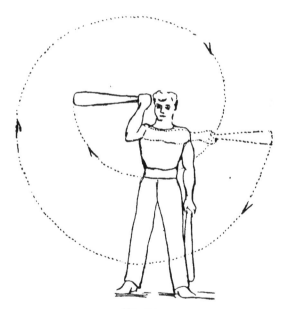

No. 192.

Exercise 152.—Same as Exercise 151 with the left club.

Exercise 153.—Change from the second series to the first series with the right club. Start as when doing Exercise 45, nearly the whole of which must be done. When half of the back circle reversed is done, and the club is pointed to the right, in the position shown by fig. 192, instead of finishing the back circle reversed, stop the swing, straighten the arm as shown in fig. 193, and swing the club

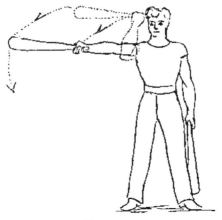

Fig. 193.

downwards, doing a front circle; thus having changed from the second series to the first.

Exercise 154.—The same as Exercise 153 done with the left club.

Exercise 155.—Changing from first to second series with both clubs at the same time; that is, Exercises 151 and 152 done together. It is also Exercise 9, fig. 66, changed into Exercise 49, fig. 109.

Start exactly as in Exercise 9, but instead of completing the back circles, change the swing as described in Exercise 151, figs. 190 and 191; both arms then get into the front circle reversed as in Exercise 49. There is no difficulty in this change if Exercises 151 and 152 have been well learnt.

Exercise 156.—Reverse Exercise 155, changing from second to first series with both clubs at the same time; that is, Exercises 153 and 154 done together.

Start exactly as in Exercise 49, fig. 109, but, instead of completing the back circles reversed, change the swing as described in Exercise 153, figs. 192 and 193 ; both clubs then fall into a front circle as in Exercise 9.

Exercise 157.—Changing in the third series the direction of the clubs from the right side to the left.

This is a very useful change in doing the third series, as it enables the performer to change from one side to the other without, apparently, stopping his clubs. This change is merely Exercises 151 and 154 done together. The right club changes as in Exercise 151, and the left club as in Exercise 154, both clubs going *together*, and doing the change *together*. This change is shown in fig. 194.

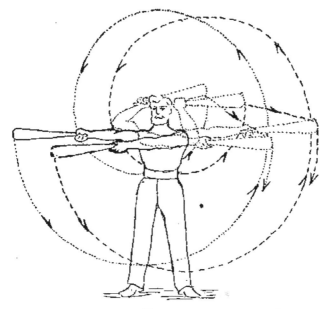

FIG. 194.

Of course the pupil must get perfect in the single changes with each arm separately before he attempts those with the two clubs together.

Exercise 158.—The same as Exercise 157, but starting to the left, so that the clubs change from the left side to the right. The right club does Exercise 153, and the left Exercise 152.

Exercise 159.—Another way of changing from the second to the first series. With the right club start with a front circle reversed; when the club reaches the right side, bend the arm, as shown in fig. 195; that is, as in beginning a back circle, stop the upward swing of the club and do a back circle, thus having changed from the second to the first series.

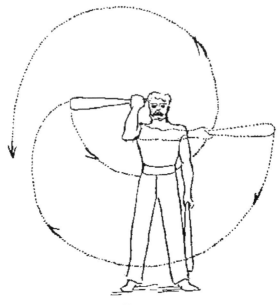

Fig. 195.

Exercise 160.—Same as Exercise 159, done with the left arm.

From the preceding changes alone, the pupil can get some very good exercises. For instance, by combining Exercises 151 and 153 together: start with the front circle—*one*, back circle—*two*, change and front circle reversed—*three*, back circle reversed—*four*, change and front circle—*one*, back circle—*two*, and so on.

Another very good exercise is combining Exercises 151 and 159, thus: front circle reversed—*one*, change and back circle (fig. 195)—*two*, front circle—*three*, back circle and change (fig. 191)—*four*.

Another exercise can also be done by alternating Exercises 155 with 156, Exercises 157 and 158. In fact, those changes, if combined together or with the other 150 exercises, can make so many different combinations that if I were to name them all a book many times larger than this one would be wanted.

Table showing the Order in which the Exercises ought to be Learnt.

The numbers refer to the corresponding numbers given to each exercise in the book. Where the name of the circle is given, it is a key exercise, and must be learnt from the description given for key exercises in Chapter I., or in Chapter III., according to the circle mentioned.

(Numbers to be read downwards.)

No. of the Exercise.	No. of the Exercise.
Front circle ... ...Right club.	Back circle ... ...Right club.
1	5
Front circle ... ..Left club.	Back circle ... ...Left club.
2	6
3	7
Front circle reversed ...Right club.	8
41	Back circle reversed ...Right club.
Front circle reversed ...Left club.	45
42	Back circle reversed ...Left club.
43	46
81	47
82	48
4	83
44	84

M

No. of the Exercise.	No. of the Exercise.
85	Front wrist circle ...Left club.
86	22
9	23
10	24
49	25
50	26
11	27
12	28
13	29
14	30
51	Front wrist circle reversed. Right club.
52	61
53	Front wrist circle reversed. Left club.
54	62
Side wrist circle ...Right club.	63
15	64
Side wrist circle ...Left club.	65
16	66
17	67
18	68
19	69
20	70
Side wrist circle reversed. Right club	87
55	88
Side wrist circle reversed. Left club.	89
56	90
57	91
58	92
59	93
60	94
Front wrist circle ...Right club.	95
21	96
	97

No. of the Exercise.	No. of the Exercise.
98	Lower back circle reversed. Right club.
99	131
100	Lower back circle reversed. Left club.
101	132
102	133
31	134
32	135
33	136
34	141
35	142
71	143
72	144
73	127
74	137
75	145
83	146
103	36
104	37
105	38
106	39
107	40
108	76
109	77
110	78
Lower back circle ...Right club.	79
121	80
Lower back circle ...Left club.	111
122	112
123	113
124	114
125	115
126	116
	117

No. of the Exercise.	No. of the Exercise.
118	150
119	151
120	152
128	153
129	154
130	155
138	156
139	157
140	158
147	59
148	160
149	

CHAPTER V.

I SHALL now give a few exercises with the clubs, which may be used to advantage, although they really come more within the range of Dumb-bells exercises and such like than of Indian Clubs proper.

However, they are very good for strengthening the muscles, besides affording a little change. With very light clubs they form a capital exercise for children, boys or girls. The number of these exercises is rather limited, as they do not lend themselves to such combinations as the more improved manner of using the clubs. The exercises that I am about to describe were mostly in use before the club exercise had arrived to the perfection it has now, and even at the present time some teachers of the old school, and most of the so-called teachers of Calisthenics and the like, still make them the mainstay of their teaching, for want of anything better. If they were to set about learning the more approved style of using the clubs, they would soon find that both the health and the enjoyment of their pupils would benefit by it. However, there is no doubt that to those unable to bear the fatigue and strain of the regular club exercise the following must prove most useful in their results if done with very light clubs.

Some might think, after going through the following exercises, that I ought to have begun instead of finishing with them. I have not done so because I was afraid that they would spoil the pupil for learning the clubs in the way I had devised for him to follow. He, knowing nothing, could be better guided as I thought best, and also better follow me; but if he had first learnt the exercises I am now going to explain he would have, no doubt, mixed them up with what I was teaching him, which would have been a drawback instead of a help, as these exercises are in no way connected with the first 160 exercises of this book.

I shall number the following exercises, thus avoiding confusion and having numbers for reference.

Be very careful as regards the position of the feet, whether close together or apart.

The starting position is holding the clubs down by the sides of the legs, unless otherwise stated.

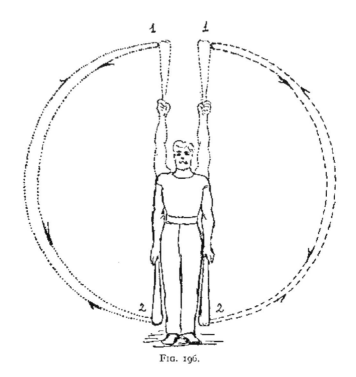

Fig. 196.

Exercise 161.—Stand feet together, heels touching one another, toes slightly apart, both clubs hanging down by the side, body perfectly erect, head well up, chest out, shoulders well down. Now with straight arms raise the clubs sideways above the head, counting—*one*—down sideways with straight arms to the starting position—*two*. Fig. 196.

Exercise 162.—Feet together, clubs at the side and position as in Exercise 161. With straight arms raise the clubs frontways above the head—*one*, down in the same way to the side—*two*. Fig. 197.

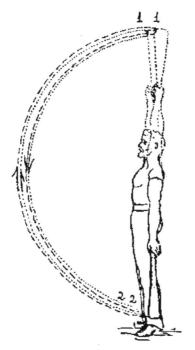

FIG. 197.

Exercise 163.—Feet together, clubs at the side. With straight arms raise the clubs sideways above the head as in Exercise 161—*one* —bringing them down frontways as in Exercise 162—*two*.

Exercise 164.—Feet together. With straight arms raise the clubs frontways above the head as in Exercise 162—*one*; bring them down sideways with straight arms as in Exercise 161—*two*.

Exercise 165.—Feet together. With straight arms raise the clubs sideways until both arms and clubs form a horizontal line—*one*; down sideways to the starting position—*two*. Fig. 198.

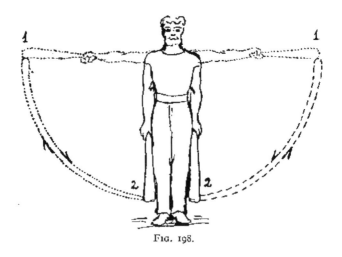

Fig. 198.

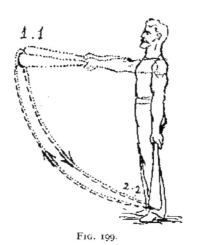

Fig. 199.

Exercise 166.—Feet together. Raise the clubs frontways with straight arms until they are in a horizontal position—*one*; down frontways—*two*. Fig. 199.

Exercise 167.—Feet together. Raise the clubs sideways until they form a horizontal line as in Exercise 165—*one*; from there bring them horizontally forward with straight arms until they are in position— one of Exercise 166, count—*two*; then bring them down frontways with straight arms as in Exercise 166, count—*three*. This exercise is shown in fig. 200.

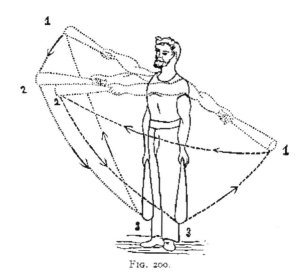

F1G. 200.

Exercise 168.—Reverse Exercise 167. Feet together; raise the clubs frontways until they are in a horizontal position as in Exercise 166, fig. 199—*one;* from that position bring them horizontally sideways in the position one of Exercise 167—*two;* then down sideways—*three.*

Exercise 169.—Same as Exercise 167, but instead of bringing the clubs down frontways, return to the sideways position, and then bring down the clubs sideways.

The exercise is done as follows :—Feet together; raise the clubs sideways to the horizontal position—*one;* bring them frontways—*two;* take them back sideways—*three;* bring them down sideways—*four.*

Exercise 170.—Raise the clubs frontways to the horizontal position—*one;* bring them sideways—*two;* back frontways—*three;* down frontways—*four.*

Exercise 171.—Raise the clubs sideways to the horizontal position —*one;* in that position, keeping the arms perfectly straight, bring the clubs, by strength of wrist, towards the forearm—*two;* then back in position one—*three;* down sideways—*four.* Fig. 201.

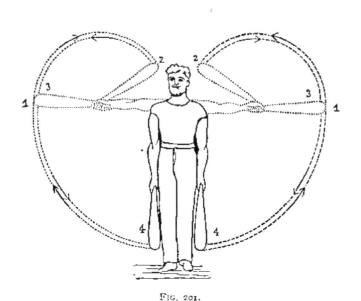

Fig. 201.

Exercise 172.—Exactly as Exercise 171, but after time *three* raise the clubs with straight arms above the head, as in Exercise 161, and count —*four;* bring the clubs down sideways again to the horizontal position— *five;* then again bring the clubs towards the forearm, as in time *two* of

Exercise 171—*six;* back to position five—*seven;* down sideways—*eight.*
Fig. 202.

Exercise 173.—The same as Exercise 171, but done frontways
instead of sideways.   Begin as in Exercise 166, fig. 199.

Exercise 174.—Same as Exercise 172 done frontways instead of
sideways.   Start as in the last exercise.

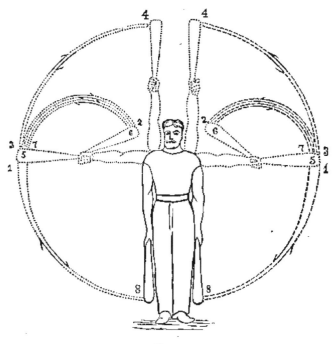

No. 202.

Exercise 175.—Hold the clubs out sideways and horizontally, as in
position of time one in fig. 201, and, keeping the arms in *that position,* do
a dozen or more consecutive wrist movements, as in Exercise 171, fig. 201,
without dropping the clubs down by the side.   Count—*one—two.* Start
counting when the clubs are up ; count—*one* when they are leaning over
the forearm and *two* when they are held out straight.

Exercise 176.—Same kind of exercise as Exercise 175, holding the clubs frontways as in Exercise 174. Same counting as Exercise 175.

Exercise 177.—Same kind of exercise as Exercise 175, but at time one the right club is extended outwards, as in time one of fig. 201, whilst the left club leans over the forearm, as in time two of fig. 201 ; thus, the ends of both clubs are pointed in the same direction—that is, towards the right; count—*one*. At—*two*, reverse the position of the clubs, both now pointing to the left. Then back towards the right, then towards the left, and so on.

Exercise 178.—Same kind of exercise as Exercise 175, but instead of moving the clubs towards the forearm and away, turn them from front to back, as in fig. 203. Start holding the clubs straight up with straight arms ; then turn them forwards—*one ;* turn them backwards—*two*, and so on. Fig. 203.

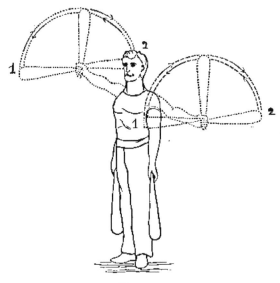

FIG. 203

Exercise 179.—Feet together. Extend the arms horizontally sideways as in time one of fig. 198; from there bring them above the head sideways with straight arms. Count—*one*; back to the horizontal position—*two*; up again—*one*, and so on.

Exercise 180.—Extend the arms horizontally frontways, as in time one of fig. 199; from there bring the clubs above the head frontways with straight arms—*one*; back to the horizontal position—*two*.

Exercise 181.—Hold the arms sideways, as in Exercise 179; from there bring them forward, exactly as in Exercise 167, time two of fig. 200. Count—*one*; then back to the first position—*two*. Again forward—*one*; back—*two*, and so on.

Exercise 182.—Exercise 179, adding the wrist motion, as in Exercise 171, fig. 201—*one—two—three—four*.

Exercise 183.—Exercise 180, with the same wrist motion, but done frontways—*one* to *four*.

Exercise 184.—Exercise 181, with the wrist motion, both at the side and forward. Time—*one* to *six*, thus: Clubs from side to front—*one*; wrist motion towards forearm—*two*; back—*three*; arms from the front to the side—*four*; wrist motion towards forearm—*five*; back—*six*; then begin again.

I shall remark here that the wrist motion of Exercise 178, fig. 203, can be done instead of the one of Exercise 171, fig. 201, wherever this last one is used. It will thus give seven new exercises. Indeed, the last 23 exercises can be combined together in various other ways, according to the fancy of the teacher or the pupil. The next exercise will enable them again to make a new set of exercises from all the 23 preceding ones.

Exercise 185.—From the starting position of Exercise 161, fig. 196, bring the clubs up by the sides as in the starting position (see fig. 13), counting—*one*; from there down again—*two*. This exercise is shown in fig. 204.

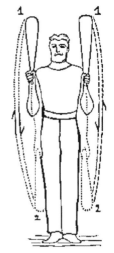

FIG. 204.

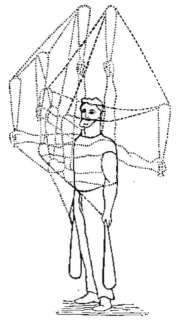

FIG. 205.

Fig. 205 shows how some of the next few exercises are to be done. It will be noticed that the clubs are held up during the exercises, as in time one of Exercise 185, fig. 204.

The numbers in the figure refer only to Exercises 186, 187, and 188. Doing those three exercises will give a perfect idea of how the others are to go. In fact, they are a mere repetition of the preceding ones with a different way of holding the clubs.

Exercise 186.—Clubs down by the side of the legs. Bring the clubs up to the side, as in Exercise 185—*one ;* above the head—*two ;* down by the side—*three ;* to the side of the legs—*four.*

Exercise 187.—Clubs down. Up by the side—*one ;* sideways with straight arms—*two ;* back to the side—*three ;* down—*four.*

Exercise 188.—Clubs down. Up by the side—*one ;* frontways, straight arms—*two ;* back to the sides—*three ;* down—*four.*

Exercise 189.—Clubs down. Up by the side—*one ;* above head —*two ;* down straight arms frontways—*three ;* to the side—*four ;* down —*five.*

Exercise 190.—Reverse Exercise 189. By the side—*one ;* frontways with straight arms—*two ;* from there with straight arms above the head—*three ;* down by the side—*four ;* down by the legs—*five.*

Exercise 191.—Up by the sides—*one ;* above head—*two ;* down straight arms sideways—*three ;* to the side—*four ;* down—*five.*

Exercise 192.—Reverse 191. Sides—*one ;* sideways straight arms —*two ;* above head—*three ;* sides—*four ;* down—*five.*

Exercise 193.—Arms out sideways, as in time three of Exercise 191, as shown in fig. 205. Keeping the arms straight bring them frontways—*one ;* back sideways with straight arms—*two.*

Exercise 194.—Arms up sideways. With straight arms bring the clubs above the head—*one ;* back with straight arms sideways—*two.*

Exercise 195.—Arms up frontways. Bring the clubs above head with straight arms—*one ;* down frontways—*two.*

Exercise 196.—Clubs down. Bring them up to the side—*one ;* both to the right in a horizontal position—*two* (as shown in time two of fig. 206) ; by the side—*three ;* both to the left (as in time one of fig. 206) —*four ;* by the side—*five ;* down—*six.*

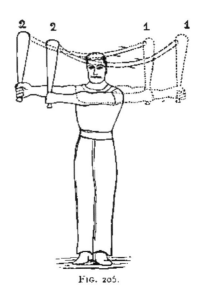

FIG. 206.

Exercise 197.—Hold the clubs to the right, as in time two of fig.
206. With straight arms bring the clubs to the left, passing them frontways—*one ;* back to the right—*two*. In this exercise the clubs are not
brought to the sides, but are simply swung from right to left and *vice versa*,
as shown in fig. 206, which represents this exercise.

Here I finish the exercises where the clubs are held up during the whole
of the exercise. I might go on giving more exercises of this description,
but I think I have shown sufficiently how to work from one exercise to
another, and I leave the pupil to find others as they may suggest themselves to him.

The few following exercises give more play to the whole body, the legs
generally taking part in them.

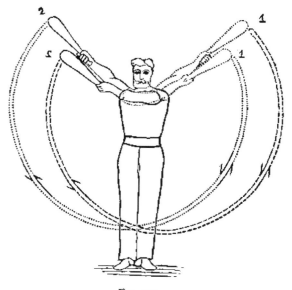

FIG. 207.

Exercise 198.—Feet together ; raise both clubs above the head to the right side, as shown in fig. 207—*one* ; then with hardly any stoppage, bring them down and up to the left side above the head—*two*. The body turns slightly towards the clubs. Fig. 207 shows this exercise.

N

Exercise 199.—Feet together. Raise quickly both clubs frontways until they are above the head, and let them hang over the shoulders, as shown by the dotted position in fig. 208, taking at the same time one step forward with the left foot; count—*one.* Bring back the clubs vigorously to the starting position, and at the same time also bring back the left foot to the side of the right—*two.* This exercise is shown in fig. 208.

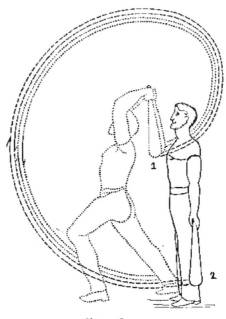

Fig. 208

Exercise 200.—Same as Exercise 199, but stepping forward with the right foot instead of the left—*one—two.*

Exercise 201.—Same as Exercise 199, but stepping alternately with the right and the left—*one—two.*

Exercise 202.—Same as Exercise 199, but stepping backwards instead of forwards with the right leg—*one—two.*

Exercise 203.—Same as Exercise 202, but stepping backwards with the left instead of the right—*one—two.*

Exercise 204.—Same as Exercise 202, but stepping backwards alternately with right and left—*one—two.*

Exercise 205.—Before beginning this exercise, first step forward with the right leg and *remain in that position* during the exercise. Swing the clubs up and down as in the preceding exercise; when this has been done about a dozen times in succession, recover to the first or starting position by bringing the right foot back to the side of the left, stopping, of course, at the same time the swinging of the clubs. Up swing—*one*; down swing—*two.*

Exercise 206.—Same as Exercise 205, but with the left foot forward—*one—two.*

Exercise 207.—Same as Exercise 198, but letting the clubs drop over the shoulders as in Exercise 199. The feet are kept together—*one —two.*

Exercise 208.—Same as Exercise 207, but instead of keeping the feet together step to the side, to the right with the right leg when the clubs are going up to the right, counting—*one*, and to the left with the left leg when the clubs are going up to the left—*two.*

Exercise 209.—Same as Exercise 207, but instead of having the feet together, place them about twenty-four inches apart from one another —not one in front of the other, but both on the same line, as in the regular club exercises; then swing the clubs to the right, facing to the right—*one*; then to the left, facing to the left—*two.* Turn on the heels, but do not move the feet off the ground.

Exercise 210.—Same kind of exercise as Exercise 205, but swinging the clubs alternately instead of together. Step forward with the right foot, raise the right club above the head, then when the right club goes down, raise the left, so that both clubs work at the same time, one going upwards whilst the other goes downwards; count—*one—two.* Do this exercise also with the left foot forward.

I shall stop here with these exercises. Out of the fifty I have described in this chapter many others can be formed, and I think I have sufficiently shown and explained how that can be done. I may also add that these exercises can be done with dumb-bells of about 1¼lb. for young children to 4lbs. for adults instead of with clubs. They can also be done without any clubs or dumb-bells by simply shutting the fists and moving the arms as indicated in the exercises, never forgetting of course to use the legs whenever they are to be used. Done this way—that is, without clubs or dumb-bells—these exercises may prove of the utmost benefit to weakly persons of either sex and of almost any age. Never jerk in any exercise—not only is it ungraceful, but it is also liable to cause a nasty jar in the joints.

CHAPTER VI.

Heavy Clubs.

IN using heavy clubs the first question is, what is the weight of the clubs to be used ?   The second question is, what exercises are to be done with heavy clubs ?

As regards the weight of the clubs it must easily be seen that what is heavy for one man may be light for another.   A man weighing 8 stone and standing barely 5 feet 6 inches can seldom use clubs of the same size or weight as a man weighing 13 stone and standing 6 feet high.   However, as a general rule, one club of 20lbs. or two of 15lbs. each are what I recommend for ordinary practice, no matter how strong the man may be. I myself use clubs weighing 80lbs. the pair, that is 40lbs. each, and I have wielded some still heavier, up to 56lbs. each, but that is quite an exception, and more for show than usual practice.   Therefore I repeat that for anyone desirous of working with heavy clubs a pair of 15lbs. each, or one of 20lbs., is quite enough.   Some supposed strong men may say, " That is not heavy," but take no notice of such remarks, as our object is to gain health as well as strength, and not to rival the modern Samsons, many of whom I have found not always strictly particular in being accurate in stating the weight of the implements they use.   By a free use of the multiplication tables they make some people believe that they are using tremendous weights, which are generally a hollow mockery. I have often seen weights or clubs of about 8 to 10lbs. mentioned as weighing from 50 to 60lbs., and sometimes more.   A man employed at one of the largest gymnastic apparatus makers in London once told me that they had succeeded in making for a professional a club of a kind of solid cork wood, quite as large as my 40 pounders, and yet weighing barely 3lbs., but which I daresay when used in public was either marked or given out to weigh 90 or 100lbs. This kind of deception is harmless enough in itself, and yet it is often the indirect cause of people inflicting on themselves life-lasting injuries by attempting to rival or excel what they happen to have seen done, without even trying to think whether what they saw could possibly be genuine or not.

To the other question, "What are the exercises to be done with heavy clubs?" I may answer, all those I have already described, and to convince the unbelievers, I shall say that with a pair of clubs of 21lbs. each I have done all the exercises in this book with the exception of twenty at the most, and these I have done with a pair of 15lbs. clubs. This ought to satisfy any enquiries on that subject, and with a pair of 15lbs. clubs, as I recommend, there ought to be no difficulty in becoming able with time and practice to accomplish all the exercises that I have mentioned above. However, I will give a table enumerating in their respective order the exercises which are best done with heavy clubs, and may prove most useful for general practice.

I must here call special attention to the proper position, and to the remarks on the same which I have made at the beginning of this book; see figs. 14 to 17.

Heavy clubs are worked in much slower time than the light ones. There should be no jerking, and everything ought to go evenly and appear as if done with the greatest ease.   I cannot do better than ask the pupil to recall all that I have said as to the way clubs must be used, as the more attention is paid to all that now, the easier the use of heavy clubs will be found.   Do not hurry, and do everything neatly ; do not attempt too much at once, but get perfect in the simplest exercises before attempting the more difficult ones.   Of course the exercises are done exactly in the same way and counting as described for the light clubs.

Table of Exercises for Heavy Clubs.

EACH EXERCISE TO BE DONE ABOUT SIX TIMES.

The numbers refer to the corresponding numbers given to each exercise in the book.

No. of the Exercise.	No. of the Exercise.	No. of the Exercise.
1	121	186
2	122	187
41	124	188
42	125	189
81	131	190
82	132	191
4	134	192
44	135	193
5	141	194
6	142	195
7	143	196
8	144	199
45	151	200
46	152	201
47	153	202
48	154	203
83	155	204
84	156	205
85	157	206
86	158	207
11	159	208
12	160	209
51	185	210
52		

Having learnt the exercises mentioned in the foregoing table, the pupil, if he can do them with great ease, may attempt whichever of the others he may most fancy, but I should recommend the following done in the order given in the general table, page 112 :—

Exercises 15 to 34
Exercises 55 ,, 74
Exercises 87 ,, 120
Exercises 145 ,, 150
Exercises 197 and 198

So far, I have mentioned exercises for one pair of clubs, but the heavy club practice consists principally and essentially of exercises with *one club only*, thus enabling the body to counterbalance the weight of the club. I have recommended a club of 20lbs. I think it is sufficient for all purposes, and, although heavier ones are often used, I shall simply repeat my former remarks as to weight.

The single heavy club can be used with both hands, but this I can hardly recommend, being ungainly, and giving a one-sided action unless the hands can be shifted at each swing. Using both hands is only good for play, and not serious useful practice.

In order to work properly with one club, it is necessary to know how to pass the club from one hand to the other. I shall explain how it is done, and I may say at once that it is very simple and easy. Following my former rule, I shall give a number to this, as an exercise.

Exercise 211.—Pass from the front circle with the right arm to the front circle reversed with the left.

Start with the right arm, holding the club in the right hand, begin a front circle. When the club is passing the right leg, take hold of the club with the left hand, letting go at the same time with the right, and without stopping the direction of the swing for one instant. There is not the slightest difficulty in this changing of hands ; it is exactly what anyone does when taking with his left hand a stick he held in his right.

Fig. 209 shows where the change is done. It must be noticed that when once in the left hand the club does a front circle reversed.

Exercise 212.—Same kind of change, but starting with the left hand and passing the club to the right. The club changes hands when passing by the left leg.

Exercise 213.—Practice changing alternately from left to right

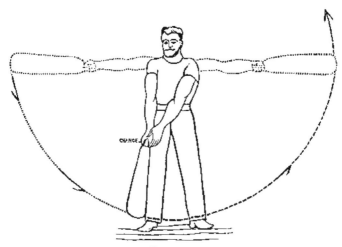

FIG. 209.

and from right to left. Start as in Exercise 211, change to the left hand, continue the swing until the club and arm are in a horizontal position, as shown in fig. 209, then stop the swing upwards, let the club come back downwards, as in Exercise 212, and pass to the right hand. The motion is like that of a pendulum.

Exercise 214.—Pass from a front circle reversed to a front circle.

Start with the right arm, doing a front circle reversed. When the arm and club pass by the left shoulder, take hold of the club with the left hand, letting go with the right, and continue the swing with the left, doing a front circle. This change is shown by fig. 210.

Exercise 215.—Same as Exercise 214, but starting with the left and passing to the right.

Exercise 216.—Change alternately from right to left and from left to right. Start as in Exercise 214, from right to left, continue the front circle with the left until the club is in the starting position of Exercise 215, stop the swing, bring the club downwards (thus doing a front circle reversed with the left), and pass to the right hand, as in Exercise 215.

It must have been noticed that the change from the front circle to the front circle reversed is done downwards when the club passes the legs (see fig. 209), and that the change from the front circle reversed to the front circle is done upwards when the club passes the head (see fig. 210).

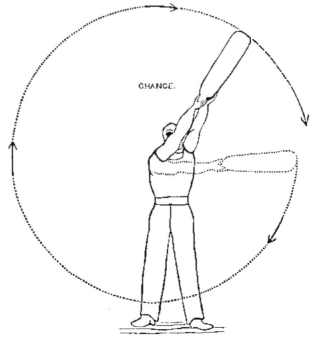

CHANCE.

FIG. 210.

Exercise 217.—This is another change, from back circle reversed with one hand to back circle with the other. Start exactly as in Exercise 45 ; do a front circle reversed and a back circle reversed with the right arm, and when this is completed, instead of extending the arm and doing a front circle reversed, bring up the left hand and take hold of the club, letting go with the right ; do not stop the swing of the club, but do a back circle with the left. Fig. 211 shows where the change is done ; the change occurs in front of the face, a little to the left.

Exercise 218.—Same as Exercise 217, but starting with the left and passing to the right, the change being done at the right side of the face.

I have now given the three principal changes for the *single* heavy

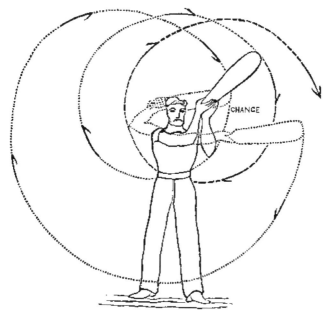

club, but those described in the light clubs are also used, and by experience and practice some others will suggest themselves. At any rate,
I may safely say that for the single club exercises the principal changes
are—for the same hand, Exercises 151 to 154, 159 and 160—from one
hand to the other, Exercises 211 to 218. I shall now give a few combinations which can be done by means of the changes.

Exercise 219.—A combination of Exercise 211 and Exercise 215,
starting with the right arm. Start and change as in Exercise 211,
continue the front circle reversed with the left and change as in Exercise
215; this change brings the club again to the right hand, as in starting. It must be noticed that the club swings in the same direction,
alternating front circle with the right and front circle reversed with the left.

Exercise 220.—Same as Exercise 219, but starting to the left; a
combination of Exercises 212 and 214.

Exercise 221.—A combination of Exercise 211 and Exercise 218.
Start and change as in Exercise 211, continue the front circle reversed
with the left, do a back circle reversed with that arm, and change to the
right, as in Exercise 218, after which the right begins again Exercise 211.

Exercise 222.—Same as Exercise 221, but starting with the left.

Exercise 223.—A combination of Exercise 151 and Exercise 214, and of Exercise 152 and Exercise 215. Do Exercise 151 (fig. 191) entirely. At the end of that exercise the right arm is doing a front circle reversed, which is the same as in the beginning of Exercise 214, therefore, after the front circle reversed, do the change of Exercise 214, which brings the club to the left hand doing a front circle, as in the beginning of Exercise 152. Do Exercise 152, after which the change as in Exercise 215, which brings the club again in the starting position of Exercise 151.

Exercise 224.—A combination of Exercise 153 and Exercise 211, and of Exercise 154 and Exercise 212. Do Exercise 153 (fig. 193) entirely. At the end of that exercise the right arm is doing a front circle, as in the beginning of Exercise 211; from that front circle do the change of Exercise 211, which brings the club to the left hand doing a front circle reversed, as in the beginning of Exercise 154. Do Exercise 154, and after that the change of Exercise 212, which brings the club to the right again, as in he sttarting position of Exercise 153.

Exercise 225.—A combination of Exercise 151 and Exercise 217, and of Exercise 152 and Exercise 218. It is exactly the same kind of exercise as Exercise 223, but using the changes of Exercise 217 and Exercise 218. Do Exercise 151 entirely, which brings the right arm in a front circle reversed, which is the beginning of Exercise 217; do that exercise and its change, which brings the club to the left, as in Exercise 152; do that exercise, after which Exercise 218 and the change, thus bringing the club again to the right.

Exercise 226.—Another combination of the exercises used in Exercise 225. For this it is preferable to start as in Exercise 217. The change of Exercise 217 is from a back circle reversed with the right to a back circle with the left. In Exercise 226, when the club is in the left doing the back circle after the change, instead of finishing that back circle and extending the arm to a front circle, as in Exercise 225, pass *at once*, from the back circle, the club over the head as in Exercise 152 (fig. 191, Exercise 151 shows this being done with the right arm). This passing the club over the head brings the club to the starting position of Exercise 218. Do the same thing again from the left to the right, which brings the club once more to the starting position of Exercise 217. It will be seen that the front circles of Exercise 151 and Exercise 152, which were used in Exercise 225, are entirely dispensed with in Exercise 226. In short, Exercise 226 runs thus: with the right front circle reversed, back circle reversed, change to the left hand; with the left hand pass over head, front circle reversed, back circle reversed, change to right hand, pass over the head with the right and begin again. This is a good exercise when well done.

Exercise 227.—Combination of Exercise 159 and Exercise 160 with Exercise 211 and Exercise 212. This exercise is simply doing Exercise 159 on the right, then passing the club to the left with the change of Exercise 211, fig. 209, then doing Exercise 160 on the left, after which repass the club to the right with the change of Exercise 212. This Exercise 227 is a great favourite with those who, whilst wishing to use a heavy club, do not care to attempt anything difficult or arduous. This exercise is extremely easy, and can be kept on for a long time with very little fatigue or straining. It must not be hurried in any way, and the club will be found to swing almost by itself, but the body must be used well as a counterpoise to the club (see fig. 16). Fig. 212 shows Exercise 227.

I should have liked to give illustrations or figures for all the changes I have described in the foregoing exercises, but I found that the various changes in the direction the club has to go would have made the figures most difficult for the reader to understand, and would have puzzled more than helped him. However, no difficulty ought to be experienced, as I have given figures of the single changes, and reference to them whilst doing the combined changes will prove quite sufficient to refresh the memory and show how the club is to go.

Exercise 228.—Combine Exercise 227 with Exercise 45.

Start with the right arm. Front circle reversed—*one;* back circle reversed—*two;* another front circle reversed—*three;* then change of swing as shown in fig. 195—*four.* The club now descends, beginning a front circle—*five;* change hands as in Exercise 227. By this change the club is now in the left hand; do a front circle reversed—*one;* back circle reversed—*two;* another front circle reversed—*three;* then change of swing as before—*four;* bringing the club in a front circle—*five;* change hands and the club is again in the right hand as in the beginning of the exercise. This is a very good and effective exercise giving play to many muscles.

Exercise 229.—Combine Exercise 227 with a lower back circle,

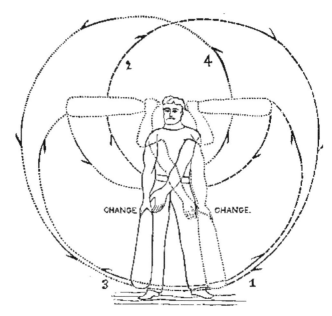

FIG. 212.

fig. 162. Start with the right arm, do a lower back circle, then change hands as in Exercise 227; do the change of swing of that exercise with the left hand, but as the club goes down, instead of doing a front circle, do a lower back circle, after which pass the club to the right hand, with which do the change of swing, thus getting again in the starting position.

Exercise 230.—Combine 227 with the lower back circle reversed. Start with the right, do a lower back circle reversed, and after that circle, when the club is in the position shown by the dotted club in fig. 162, bend the right arm and do the change of swing as in fig. 212 then downwards and pass the club to the left hand, following this change by a lower back circle reversed with the left, after which change the swing as before, then change hands, being again at the starting point.

Many more exercises can be done by combinations, but I think I have given enough for all practical purposes; others will suggest themselves to the advanced performer.

With the heavy clubs there are also done what are termed *slow exercises*, or feats of strength. I shall just name a few for those who care to practice them. This kind of exercise can be done with one club, doing the exercise first with one hand, then with the other; or they can be done with both clubs at the same time. They must be done very slowly, and entirely by muscular power. Many people in doing so-called feats of strength in gymnastics go very slowly over the easy portion of the exercise, but when at the difficult part they get over it by a quick jerk; this deceives the uninitiated; but after all they are only cheating themselves as well. So it is with the slow club exercises.

In fig. 213 I have shown the position of a few of the following exercises. All these exercises ought to be done first with a single club and afterwards with both.

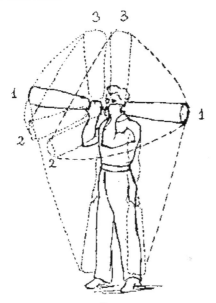

FIG. 213.

Exercise 231.—Bring the right club slowly to the position one of fig. 213, then slowly down to the starting point.

Exercise 232.—Same with the left club.

Exercise 233.—Bring the right club up slowly as before to position one ; from that position bring it slowly to position two of fig. 213 ; then back to position one, and down slowly.

Exercise 234.—Same with the left club.

Exercise 235.—Right club slowly up to position one, from there slowly up to position three, fig. 213, back slowly to position one, and down.

Exercise 236.—Same with the left.

Exercise 237.—Right club slowly up to position 1 ; from there to position 3, then to position 2, back again to position 1, then to position 2, back to position 3, down to position 1, then down. All must be done slowly.

Exercise 238.—Same with the left.

This last exercise is capital for both clubs ; in fact, Exercises 231 to 238 should be done with both clubs *together* as well as with one. The few foregoing slow exercises can be greatly varied, as the pupil can easily see for himself.

Exercise 239.—This exercise is done with both clubs. Hold the clubs as shown in fig. 214, and whilst in that position turn them round one another as indicated by the dotted circles in fig. 214. This exercise

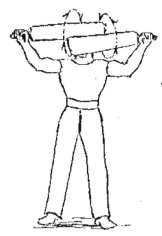

Fig. 214.

is to be done first with the clubs going towards the head, as shown by the arrows of the circles in fig. 214. Do this several times, then reverse the motion, the clubs going away from the head.   The clubs must go round one another slowly.

Exercise 240.—This is also done with both clubs.   Bring them slowly up to position one of fig. 215, holding them with straight arms, and from there bring them forward slowly with straight arms to position two, then back slowly with straight arms to position one, then slowly down.

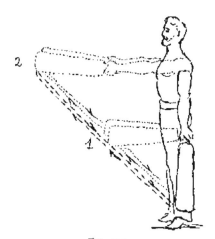

FIG. 215.

I shall here conclude the heavy clubs exercises, though I might have described many more, those I have given here being capable of combining in almost endless variations.

I may just add that there are many juggling tricks to be done with the clubs, but I do not approve of them for the light clubs, as I consider that they belong more to professional bottle juggling than to Indian Club exercises.   Juggling with the heavy clubs has more *raison d'etre* owing to the weight of the clubs, but even then it belongs more to exhibition work than to genuine and beneficial club exercise.   Juggling is by no means difficult, requiring simply a very quick eye, great steadiness, and a great amount of practice, but above all an utter disregard to the hands,

O

thumbs, and fingers, which may sometimes get seriously injured.
Juggling is very taking with the public, and my own experience is that it
seems to please them more than any of the most arduous or clever combinations.   However, I do not think it necessary to introduce juggling
here, as anyone wishing to practise it will soon find how it is done, and if
the club is heavy, how it feels.

APPENDIX.

STRENGTH AND STRONG MEN.

I HAVE always found that tales of marvellous strength have a kind of fascination to most people engaged in athletics, and more especially to gymnasts. For the delectation of those of my readers who may be thus inclined, I shall give here a few instances of wonders of strength, mentioning them as briefly as possible.

Strength is not a gift possessed by everyone; some people are naturally strong, others acquire strength by work and practice. As regards strength in ordinary men, we generally find that the bigger the man the stronger he is; it is simply a question of weight against weight (by weight I do not mean fat). Take, for instance, two men wrestling together, one weighing 150lbs. and the other 200lbs; the lighter man would have to lift 200lbs., that is 50lbs. over his own weight, or, in other words, 1⅓rd of himself; whereas the heavier man, having to lift only 150lbs., or 50lbs. less than his own weight, would only be lifting ¾ of his weight. The lighter man would therefore have to put out ⅝ths more strength than the heavier one, that is to say, almost as much again. From this it is evident that with men of equal strength in proportion to their size the biggest ought to be the strongest; and it is worthy of remark that most of the men noted for their extraordinary strength were of great size. Again, supposing that the two men I have instanced above are lifting weights, say 100lbs. each, it stands to reason that if the lighter man lifts his weight as well as the heavier one does his, he, the lighter man, must be the strongest of the two, as he lifts ⅔rds of his own weight, whereas the heavier man only lifts ½ of his; the heavier man to be as strong as the lighter one would have to lift 133lbs.

Bodily strength does not, however, depend only on the size of the body or of the muscles, but also on the solidity of the bones, and the conformation of the muscles, on their harmony, and above all, on the impulse received from the brain. This impulse or energy has a real influence on the muscular power; it is, so to speak, the hidden force. This explains the extraordinary strength sometimes displayed by men of thin appearance, whilst other men, with thick and fleshy bodies, are far from possessing the power one would expect from their bulk. This brain-produced energy is again apparent by the extraordinary increase of power which is often derived from excitement, such as that created by applause, music, or anything else acting on the senses. However, to obtain perfect bodily strength it is necessary to add to this brain energy a good, sound, muscular development equally distributed over the body. A perfect athlete ought to be able to do all kinds of exercises equally well. Such a man is represented in an exaggerated form by the statue of the Farnese Hercules; here the sculptor has endeavoured to represent a man in whose power it was to do everything, from carrying the heaviest load to running down the fleetest animals. For mere brute strength it is certain that bulk, height and weight have the advantage.

In all countries and at all times there have been men of extraordinary strength, some of them possessing a muscular power so far beyond belief that one cannot help thinking that some exaggeration must have cropped up in the records which have reached us of their doings.

Of the wonderful athletes of all ages, Milo, of Cretone, is perhaps the most known. He once ran a mile with an ox on his shoulders; then, with a blow of his fist, he killed the beast, and ate it in one day. The latter exploit, which can hardly be called a feat of strength (it is more a feat of digestion), is referred to in the following lines, which until recently could be seen over the doorway of the Queen's Hotel, facing the General Post Office, Aldersgate : —

> Milo the Cretonian
> An ox slew with his fist,
> And ate it up at one meal—
> Ye gods! what a glorious twist!

The strongest man could not take from Milo a pomegranate which he held between his two fingers, although a woman he loved is said to have done it. He could break, by contracting his veins and muscles, a cord tied round his forehead. One day, being in a house with some pupils of Pythagoras, the ceiling threatened to fall in, but Milo supported the column on which it rested, thus giving his friends time to escape. His death is well known; he tried to tear asunder the trunk of a tree, but his hands got pinched in the wood, and being unable to disengage them he perished, devoured by wild beasts.

Polydamas, of Thessalia, was a man of extraordinary strength and stature. As Hercules had done, he alone, without arms, killed an enormous lion that was devastating the valleys of Mount Olympus. With one hand Polydamas could hold back a chariot drawn by two horses. He could break the trunk of a tree as anyone would break a small stick. The King of Persia, Darius I., wishing to witness the feats of this marvellous man, called him to his court; he opposed to him three of the strongest men of his army. Polydamas killed the three by simply giving them a slap on the ears; he was going to slap the face of a few more, when the king, satisfied, stopped him. One day he seized a bull by one of its hind feet, and the animal did not escape until it had left its hoof in Polydamas's hand. Like Milo, he died through over confidence in his strength. He attempted to support a mass of rock that had given way, but he got buried under it and died.

Theagenes, of Thasos, who, with a body like that of Apollo and the strength of Hercules, surpassed all his rivals in all kinds of exercises, won over fourteen hundred prizes.

Eurybate, Chilo, Euthymus and Astydamas won also renown as wonderful athletes.

The strength of Samson is too well known to need description here.

The Roman Emperor Caius Julius Verus Maximus was a marvel of strength, being able to squeeze the hardest stone to powder with his fingers. He was upwards of eight feet in height, and his wife's bracelet could serve him as a ring.

Salvius, of Rome, could walk up a ladder carrying 200lbs. on his shoulders, 200lbs. in his hands, and 200lbs. fastened to his feet.

Athanatus could run round the arena carrying 500lbs. on his shoulders and 500lbs. fastened to his feet.

Iccus could hold the most furious bull and tear away its horns as easily as one would pull up radishes.

Scanderberg, King of Albania, who lived in the 15th century, was reputed the strongest man of his time. He was a man of great stature, and the power of his arm was such that he thought nothing of cutting two men in half with one single blow of his sword.

Francis of Vivonne, Lord of Chasteigneraye, who lived at the court of Francis I. of France, could stop a bull by seizing it by the horns.

The Emperor Charlemagne, who stood eight feet high, could hold at arm's length a knight in full armour.

Ernaulton, of Spain, possessed wonderful strength. On Christmas Day, 1388, being with several nobles in the upper rooms of a castle, the host complained of the fire burning low; hearing this, Ernaulton, who had seen through the window some asses going by laden with wood, went out, seized one of the asses, and swinging it, together with its burden, upon his shoulders, mounted twenty-four steps to the room where the nobles were, and playfully threw wood and ass on the fire.

Louis de Boufflers, who lived in the 16th century, could break a bar of iron with his hands. The strongest man could not take from him a ball which he held between his thumb and first finger. While standing up with no support whatever, four strong soldiers could not move him; he remained as firm as a rock. Sometimes he amused himself by taking on his shoulders his own horse fully harnessed, and with that heavy load he promenaded the public square, to the great delight of the inhabitants.

At about the same period there lived a Spaniard named Piedro who could break the strongest handcuffs that could be put round his wrists. He folded his arms on his chest, and ten men pulling in different directions with ropes could not unfold them.

Also in the sixteenth century there lived another remarkably strong man, a major named Barsabas. One day he took up an anvil weighing 500lbs., and hid it under his cloak. Often, to amuse his comrades, he went through the rifle drill with a cannon. He could crush between his fingers the limbs of big animals. One day, seeing a crowd looking at an enormous dancing bear, he offered to wrestle with the animal. The major threw the bear down several times, and, judging it unworthy of further struggle, slew the animal with his fist, and carried it away on his shoulders, amidst the cheers of the crowd. Another day, seeing several officers of his regiment surrounded by an angry crowd, he ran to them, knocking people down right and left, as a child does with a pack of cards. The crowd, exasperated, turned round on him, but, seizing two of his assailants, one with each hand, he used them as clubs on the crowd, who, astonished at this extraordinary display of strength, quickly drew back. Once he squeezed to pulp the hand of a man who wanted to fight him.

Barsabas's sister was also remarkable for her strength. Some burglars entered a convent where she was ; she threw one out of the window, and killed two others with a pillar she tore down and used as a club.

Augustus II., Elector of Saxony, was a man of great strength ; he could carry a man in his open hand. One night he quietly threw out of a window a monk who paraded his palace pretending to be a ghost.

Augustus's son, the famous Maurice, Maréchal de Saxe, who commanded the French at Fontenay, was also a marvel of strength. On one occasion he twisted with his fingers only a long nail into a corkscrew, with which he drew the cork of half-a-dozen bottles. He could break with his hands the strongest horseshoe. One day when in London he had a row with a dustman, when he seized the man by the head, and throwing him up in the air, let him drop right in the middle of his own dust cart. The only opponent who succeeded in resisting him was a woman, a Mdlle. Gauthier, an actress. Maurice tried with her to see who could put down the other's wrist, and after a long struggle he won, but with the greatest difficulty. The power of Mdlle. Gauthier's arm was far beyond the common, and with her fingers she could roll up silver plate as easily as anyone would paper.

Thomas Topham, born in London in 1710, was a man possessed of extraordinary strength. He once lifted three casks filled with water, and weighing in all 1,836lbs. He is said to have had the combined strength of twelve men. He could bend a stout bar of iron by holding the two ends with his hands, placing the middle of the bar behind his neck and bringing the two ends forward. He could also undo what he had done, that is, straightening the bar again, a much more difficult feat. Once, having some words with a neighbour, he took an iron spit and twisted it round the man's neck with as much ease as if it had been a handkerchief. He could roll up a pewter dish, weighing 7lbs., with his hands as if it had been a piece of paper; he could also squeeze together a pewter quart pot whilst holding it at arm's length. He could crack cocoanuts as easily as anyone would crack hazel nuts; break a broomstick of the largest size by striking it against his bare arm; lift two hogsheads of water; lift his horse over a turnpike gate; carry the beam of a house as a soldier would his rifle; lift two hundredweights with his little finger over his head. He broke a rope fastened to the ground that would sustain twenty hundredweight, and lifted an oak table, six feet long, with his teeth, though half a hundredweight was hung at the extremity. With one hand he raised a man who weighed twenty-seven stone. Once, seeing a watchman asleep in his box, he carried away both man and box a long distance. It is said of him that, having been placed on some duty at the entrance gate of a racecourse, he refused to allow a four-horse coach to go through; on the driver whipping his horses and attempting to pass, Topham took hold of the hind wheels of the coach and upset it and its occupants into the roadway. Topham, who kept a public-house in Islington, had a wife who quarrelled with him to such an extent that she drove him to commit suicide. Hercules, Samson, Milo, and many other wonders of bodily strength had to give way to a woman; so did Topham, apparently.

At about the same time as Topham, there lived another wonderfully strong man, Richard Joy, whose feats may possibly have got mixed in records with those of Topham. Richard Joy was already renowned for his marvellous strength before Topham was born. He was commonly known as the Kentish Samson, and the strong man of Kent; among other things, he could cope successfully against any powerful horse, lift a ton weight, and snap a rope that bore 35 cwt. without breaking, the latter being far more extraordinary than Topham's similar feat. He was drowned in a smuggling expedition some ten years before Topham's death, and is buried in the churchyard of St. Peter's Church, near Broadstairs; his tombstone bears the following inscription :—

> Herculean hero, famed for strength,
> At last lies here his breadth and length ;
> See how the mighty man is fallen—
> To death the strong and weak are all one ;
> And the same judgment doth befall
> Goliath great as David small.

Joy was taken to court in the reign of William and Mary to exhibit his strength before the King and nobility.

Tom Johnson, who was champion boxer of England in 1785, could lift a sack of wheat with one hand and swing it round his head.

The sailors of Constantinople still speak of a Greek who could bend an anchor with his hands only.

The brothers Rousselle, nicknamed "Hercules du Nord," exhibited wonderful muscular power. The eldest could jump a great height (some records say ten feet), with a weight of 50lbs. fastened to his feet, and a similar weight in each hand. Standing on a chair and bending himself backwards, he could with his teeth lift from the ground a weight of 500lbs. He could lift on his shoulders a table with 1,500lbs. on it. The brothers Rousselle acquired their extraordinary strength by constant practice and careful living.

A man named Eckenberg could lift a gun weighing 2,500lbs. Two of the strongest men could not take from him a stick he held with one hand.

An Englishman is said to have held back with a rope fastened round his loins two horses urged on with a whip.

A Scotchman, said to be the last of the Stuarts, was also possessed with extraordinary strength, from which circumstance he got the bye-name of Jemmy Strength. Among other feats he could carry a twenty-four pounder cannon, and had been known to lift a cart-load of hay, weighing a ton-and-a-half, upon his back. Many a time he took up a jackass, and, carrying it on his shoulders, walked through the toll-gate.

Jonathan Fowler, an American, once walked out knee-deep through the mud and filth of a sea-shore at low tide to a shark left by the retiring waters, shouldered it, and brought it alive on his back to the shore. The shark weighed five hundred pounds, quite a load, considering that it was not the most portable of articles, and that the man had to wade through mud.

A Belgian giant could stand up under two tons.

Dr. Winship, a well-known American, can raise from the ground 1,400lbs.

A seaman on board the celebrated cruiser, the "Alabama," a Scotchman named Gill, could lift a man at arm's length with one hand.   P

Abraham Lincoln, the United States President, was a man of great strength. He could with one blow bury an axe in the trunk of a tree deeper than any other man, and he is said to have thrown across the roadway a pigeon-house weighing upwards of 600lbs.

FINIS.

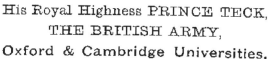
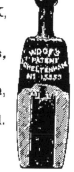

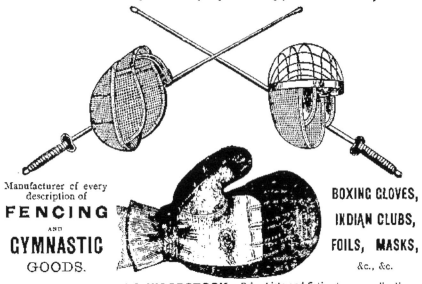
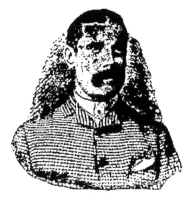

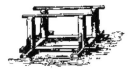

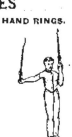

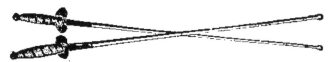

EXTRACTS OF UNSOLICITED PRESS OPINIONS

OF A FEW OF

Mr. E. F. LEMAIRE'S PERFORMANCES.

————>•◄————

" The ' King of Clubs,' Mr. E. F. Lemaire, is rightly named, seeing that he has such perfect control over those ponderous playthings."—*Graphic*.

" In the open clubs the spectators had a great treat. Among the competitors was E. F. Lemaire, of the German Gymnastic Club, London, and the display of skill and strength that he exhibited was something marvellous. His gracefulness with the light clubs, and his strength with the heavy ones, was wonderful. He wielded with dexterity and ease clubs weighing 8olbs. the pair. He was awarded the first prize."—*Yorkshire Post*.

" We must signal for special praise . . . . and the Indian Club Exercise of Mr. Lemaire."—*Daily Telegraph*.

" An elegant and muscular illustration of the Indian Club Exercise by Mr. Lemaire (G.G.S.) with 22lb., 33lb. and 44lb. clubs drew down immense applause."—*Morning Advertiser*.

" Mr. Lemaire executed some marvellous feats with the Indian Clubs, which drew down well-deserved marks of approbation."—*Hour*.

" But it was Mr. Lemaire's feats that were most admired and the most remarkable. He first manipulated with comparatively small clubs with the greatest dexterity, introducing all the most difficult evolutions. Then he operated with clubs each weighing 20lbs.; then with apparently the same ease repeated the movements with clubs each weighing 40lbs.; and afterwards, mounting a pedestal, wielded fifteen-pounders, each of which was 5ft. 7½in. in length. He received an enthusiastic *encore*."—*Yorkshire Post*.

" The Club Exercise elicited loud applause from the spectators, notably the masterly manner in which Mr. Lemaire twisted and whirled clubs weighing 22lbs., 33lbs and 44lbs. a-piece."—*Daily News*.

" The Club Exercise put all one's ordinary notions as to the wielding of clubs to flight, especially when Mr. Lemaire, after swinging about in every direction and at every kind of angle a forty-pounder, took two forty-pounders and used them with as great ease as if they had been a pair of walking-sticks."—*Standard*.

" This graceful and muscle-developing branch of athletics was done in a masterly manner, Lemaire receiving tremendous rounds of applause for his fine handling of two 40lb. clubs."—*Referee*.

" This part of the programme was a great success, and the clever wielder was greeted with great applause."—*Another Brighton Paper*.

" After . . . came one of the treats of the evening, Mr. E. F. Lemaire going through the Indian Club Exercise with 10lb., 40lb., and 8olb. pairs in a manner that excited great admiration and secured him a recall."—*Brighton Paper*.

" Mr. Lemaire is very clever with the clubs, and can manipulate two 40lbs. with grace and ease."—*Athletic World*.

" Mr. E. F. Lemaire, who was a winner in a great club competition at Leeds, went through some wonderful feats last night."—*Daily News*.

" Mr. Lemaire (G.G.S.) now varied the programme agreeably with a series of difficult exercises with the Indian Clubs. The entertainment was well worthy the attention bestowed upon it, and at the close the spectators gave the clever wielder a most enthusiastic reception."—*Sporting Life*.

" Nor did the efforts of that modern Hercules, E. F. Lemaire, with light and heavy clubs, pass unnoticed."—*Sportsman*.

" Mr. E. F. Lemaire showed some wonderful evolutions with the light and heavy clubs."

" In the use of the clubs Mr. Lemaire wielded with ease a pair of mighty weapons, which looked as if they had been borrowed from our tall friend Blunderbore in the pantomime. They weighed 40lbs. each, but Mr. Lemaire whirled them round his head as easily as if each had been a feather."—

" Mr. E. F. Lemaire, as usual, went gracefully through his marvellous feats with Indian Clubs of various weights."—

" The lion's share of applause was carried off by Mr. Lemaire, who first mounted a kind of rostrum, performed with a pair of clubs, each 5ft. 7½in in length and 15lbs. weight, and subsequently with clubs of 33lbs. and 44lbs. weight."—

" Mr Lemaire gave the novel solo of manipulating a pair of clubs upwards of 6ft. in length."—

" Loud and prolonged cheering greeted Mr. E. F. Lemaire, ot the German Gymnastic Society, who wielded heavy clubs with marvellous skill and dexterity."—

" The easy manner in which Mr. Lemaire (of Clapham Hall Gymnasium) whirled about gigantic clubs to the strains of music caused much astonishment and applause."—

" Mr. Lemaire astonished the spectators with his handling of two gigantic clubs weighing 40lbs. each."—

" The stage was now given up to Mr. E. F. Lemaire, who proceeded to show the facility with which he could wield Indian Clubs. He used clubs of 10lbs., 44lbs., and 80lbs. weight per pair, and the celerity with which he flourished them in all directions was something surprising."—

" Mr. Lemaire did what he liked with Indian Clubs of all weights, giving a remarkable exhibition of agility and strength."—

" That accomplished wielder of clubs, Mr. E. F. Lemaire, gave a most finished display, winding up with two 40lbs. clubs, which he swung with a considerable amount of ease and grace."—

" Clubs in the hands of that well-known amateur, Mr. E. F. Lemaire, diversified the entertainment, and it is almost needless to record that his display elicited the applause of the entire company."—

" Mr. E. F. Lemaire gave a fine exhibition of strength by the use of four sets of Indian Clubs, graduating from 10lbs. to 80lbs. per pair, and the latter he seemed to use with far less exertion than with the lighter weighted ones, and he certainly is a marvel of strength."—

" Inasmuch as Mr. E. F. Lemaire was the exponent, it is needless to say that the exposition was of the very best class."—

" Mr. E. F. Lemaire gave a fine display with the 10lb. to 80lb. Indian Clubs, retiring at the close of his show amidst a well-merited shower of applause, which was kept up until Mr. Lemaire re-appeared and bowed his acknowledgments."—

" At the conclusion of this contest Mr. E. F. Lemaire gave a wonderful exhibition of what could be done with Indian Clubs. A more graceful exercise it would be difficult to imagine, and Mr. Lemaire swings a pair weighing 40lbs. each almost as easily as the lighter ones."

" Cheers greeted the announcement of clubs by Mr. E. F. Lemaire, and those present were treated to a very excellent display, his cleverness being much admired, and on his retirement he met with a great ovation."—

" E. F. Lemaire then went through the Indian Club Exercise in a manner that made his name famous years ago."—

" Mr. E. F. Lemaire (the G.G.S. strong man) showed what he could do with Indian Clubs—weighing 80lbs. per pair—and weights weighing 56lbs. and 101lbs."—

(And many others.)